COMPUTATIONAL TECHNOLOGY FOR EFFECTIVE HEALTH CARE

IMMEDIATE STEPS AND STRATEGIC DIRECTIONS

William W. Stead and Herbert S. Lin, *Editors*

Committee on Engaging the Computer Science Research Community in Health Care Informatics

Computer Science and Telecommunications Board

Division on Engineering and Physical Sciences

NATIONAL RESEARCH COUNCIL
OF THE NATIONAL ACADEMIES

THE NATIONAL ACADEMIES PRESS
Washington, D.C.
www.nap.edu

THE NATIONAL ACADEMIES PRESS   500 Fifth Street, N.W.   Washington, DC 20001

NOTICE: The project that is the subject of this report was approved by the Governing Board of the National Research Council, whose members are drawn from the councils of the National Academy of Sciences, the National Academy of Engineering, and the Institute of Medicine. The members of the committee responsible for the report were chosen for their special competences and with regard for appropriate balance.

Support for this project was provided by the National Library of Medicine and the National Institute of Biomedical Imaging and Bioengineering, National Institutes of Health (Award Number N01-OD-04-2139, Task Order 182); the National Science Foundation (Award Number CNS-0638373); the Vanderbilt University Medical Center; Partners HealthCare System; the Robert Wood Johnson Foundation (Award Number 59392); and the Commonwealth Fund (Award Number 20070083). Any opinions expressed in this material are those of the authors and do not necessarily reflect the views of the agencies and organizations that provided support for the project.

International Standard Book Number 13:   978-0-309-13050-9
International Standard Book Number 10:   0-309-13050-6

Library of Congress Control Number: 2009921035

Copies of this report are available from:

The National Academies Press
500 Fifth Street, N.W., Lockbox 285
Washington, DC 20055
800/624-6242
202/334-3313 (in the Washington metropolitan area)
http://www.nap.edu

THE NATIONAL ACADEMIES
Advisers to the Nation on Science, Engineering, and Medicine

The **National Academy of Sciences** is a private, nonprofit, self-perpetuating society of distinguished scholars engaged in scientific and engineering research, dedicated to the furtherance of science and technology and to their use for the general welfare. Upon the authority of the charter granted to it by the Congress in 1863, the Academy has a mandate that requires it to advise the federal government on scientific and technical matters. Dr. Ralph J. Cicerone is president of the National Academy of Sciences.

The **National Academy of Engineering** was established in 1964, under the charter of the National Academy of Sciences, as a parallel organization of outstanding engineers. It is autonomous in its administration and in the selection of its members, sharing with the National Academy of Sciences the responsibility for advising the federal government. The National Academy of Engineering also sponsors engineering programs aimed at meeting national needs, encourages education and research, and recognizes the superior achievements of engineers. Dr. Charles M. Vest is president of the National Academy of Engineering.

The **Institute of Medicine** was established in 1970 by the National Academy of Sciences to secure the services of eminent members of appropriate professions in the examination of policy matters pertaining to the health of the public. The Institute acts under the responsibility given to the National Academy of Sciences by its congressional charter to be an adviser to the federal government and, upon its own initiative, to identify issues of medical care, research, and education. Dr. Harvey V. Fineberg is president of the Institute of Medicine.

The **National Research Council** was organized by the National Academy of Sciences in 1916 to associate the broad community of science and technology with the Academy's purposes of furthering knowledge and advising the federal government. Functioning in accordance with general policies determined by the Academy, the Council has become the principal operating agency of both the National Academy of Sciences and the National Academy of Engineering in providing services to the government, the public, and the scientific and engineering communities. The Council is administered jointly by both Academies and the Institute of Medicine. Dr. Ralph J. Cicerone and Dr. Charles M. Vest are chair and vice chair, respectively, of the National Research Council.

www.national-academies.org

Preface

It is essentially axiomatic that modern health care is an information- and knowledge-intensive enterprise.[1] The information collected in health care includes—among other things—medical records of individual patients (both paper and electronic, spread across many different health care organizations), laboratory test results, information about treatment protocols and drug interactions, and a variety of financial and administrative information. Knowledge resides in the published medical literature, in the higher-order cognitive processes of individual clinicians and care providers, and in the processes of health care organizations that facilitate the provision of care.

Whereas the practices of 20th century health care were based largely on paper, there is now a broad consensus that realizing an improved 21st century vision of health care will require intensive use of information technology to acquire, manage, analyze, and disseminate health care information and knowledge. Accordingly, the Administration and Congress have been moving to encourage the adoption, connectivity, and interoperability of health care information technology. President George W. Bush called for nationwide use of electronic medical records by 2014,[2]

---

[1]Institute of Medicine and National Academy of Engineering, *Building a Better Delivery System: A New Engineering/Health Care Partnership*, The National Academies Press, Washington, D.C., 2005, available at http://www.nap.edu/catalog.php?record_id=11378.

[2]Commission on Systemic Interoperability, *Ending the Document Game*, U.S. Government Printing Office, Washington, D.C., 2005, available at http://endingthedocumentgame.gov/.

and the Department of Health and Human Services (HHS) is involved in various aspects of achieving this goal.[3]

The National Library of Medicine launched this study to support the engagement of individuals from the computer science research community in meeting two challenges posed by health care information technology: identifying how today's computer science-based methodologies and approaches might be applied more effectively to health care, and explicating how the limitations in these methodologies and approaches might be overcome through additional research and development.

The study described in this report was conducted by an interdisciplinary committee of experts in biomedical informatics, computer science and information technology (including databases, security, networking, human-computer interaction, and large-scale system deployments), and health care providers (e.g., physicians who have worked with information technologies). Appendix A provides brief biographical information on the members and the staff of the Committee on Engaging the Computer Science Research Community in Health Care Informatics.

The committee's work focused primarily on understanding the nature and impact of the information technology investments made by major health care organizations. By design, the committee's effort was both time- and resource-limited, and thus the primary function of this report is to lay the groundwork for future efforts that can explore in a second phase some of the identified questions and issues in greater detail. Perhaps most importantly, this study does not touch, except in the most peripheral way, on a myriad of complex social, political, and economic issues that complicate the task of health care reform.

For example, although this report emphasizes the role of the clinician, there are other important decision makers in the health care system, including patients, family caregivers, and other health care professionals, whose health care information technology needs the report addresses only peripherally. Similarly, although the data-gathering efforts of the committee were focused primarily on major health care organizations, the majority of health care is delivered in small-practice settings (of two to five physicians) that lack significant organizational support. These omissions do not diminish the significance of the committee's efforts and recommendations, although they do point to the need for more work to understand health care information technology (IT) needs more thoroughly in the areas that the committee did not examine carefully.

---

[3]Institute of Medicine, *Opportunities for Coordination and Clarity to Advance the National Health Information Agenda*, The National Academies Press, Washington, D.C., 2007, available at http://www.nap.edu/catalog.php?record_id=12048.

Other important issues omitted in this report that are worthy of serious attention in follow-on reports include the explicit inclusion of instruction in health/biomedical informatics and health care IT in various forms of health care education (e.g., medical and nursing school curricula); legal and cultural barriers to sharing information among various care providers; the development of a strategic plan or roadmap that articulates the strengths, weaknesses, opportunities, and threats to the development of health care IT; standards-development processes in the health care IT industry that might facilitate interoperability; and issues related to personal health records for use by patients, the relationship of education in computer science to health care and biomedical informatics (and vice versa), and organizational support for health care providers that operate on a small scale.

The evidentiary basis for this study involved several threads. The primary observational evidence was derived from committee site visits to eight medical centers around the country (Appendix B provides the agendas for the site visits that the committee conducted). Obviously, a comprehensive view of the current state of the art in the nation's health care information technology cannot be derived from eight site visits—thus, the organizations visited must be regarded as a sampling of the state of practice throughout the country. Care was taken to ensure that the site visits were to medical centers that varied along important dimensions: governance and ownership (government-operated, non-profit, for-profit), academic and community, and in-house technology development and vendor-supplied technology. The centers visited shared one characteristic—for the most part, they were widely acknowledged to be leaders in the use of IT for health care. This choice was made because the committee felt that many of the important innovations and achievements for health care IT would be found in organizations thought to be leaders in the field.

The findings from the site visits are presented in Appendix C as a table of observations, consequences, and opportunities for action. The observations are de-identified generalizations of detail from multiple sites. The consequences and opportunities for action reflect the committee's judgment. In the main text of the committee's report, observations from site visits are cross-referenced where appropriate with the notation $CxOy$. Cx refers to Category x of the committee's observations as grouped in Table C.1 (which lists six categories of observations), and Oy refers to a particular observation as numbered in Table C.1 (which includes a total of 25 observations).

The findings from the site visits were combined with other evidentiary threads:

- *Previous work of the Institute of Medicine (IOM) and the National Academy of Engineering.* Rather than starting from scratch, the committee adopted as a point of departure for its work the IOM series "Crossing the Quality Chasm"—a vision of 21st century health care that is safe, effective, patient-centered, timely, efficient, and equitable.
- *Selective literature review.* In many instances in this report, a claim is made that is based not on direct observation but rather on one or more papers in the scientific literature.
- *Committee expertise.* The committee included a number of individuals with substantial clinical and business expertise in medical centers similar to those visited by the committee and other similar settings. Experiences from these individuals were added to this report as needed.

Eight site visits cannot support development of a statistically significant set of examples and illustrations—nevertheless, the committee believes that its observations and conclusions meet the more important test of substantive significance, especially since they arose as a result of visits to organizations regarded as among the best in the country in applying IT to solve health care problems.

Finally, although the committee's charge (Box P.1) calls attention to the computer science research community, the health/biomedical informatics research community is also a key player for doing the necessary research. The field of health/biomedical informatics emerged from medical informatics, which was described in 1990 by Greenes and Shortliffe as "the field that concerns itself with the cognitive, information processing, and communication tasks of medical practice, education, and research, including the information science and the technology to support these tasks."[4] "Health informatics" and "biomedical informatics" are more recent terms that acknowledge the increasing importance of informatics for aspects of health beyond medicine and for the basic biological sciences in medicine.

Computer science as a discipline does not subsume health/biomedical informatics, although computer scientists can and do make major contributions to that field. Health/biomedical informatics is more than medical computer science, drawing also on the decision, cognitive, and information sciences as well as engineering, organizational theory, and sociology

---

[4]Robert Greenes and Edward H. Shortliffe, "Medical Informatics: An Emerging Academic Discipline and Institutional Priority," *Journal of the American Medical Association* 263(8):1114-1120, 1990.

Box P.1 Study Statement of Task

The Computer Science and Telecommunications Board will conduct a 2-phase study to examine information technology (IT) problems faced by the health care system in realizing the emerging vision of patient-centered, evidence-based, efficient health care using electronic health records and other IT. The study will focus on the foundation issue of the electronic health record.

In phase 1, the committee will conduct a series of site visits to a variety of health care delivery sites. A short (roughly 5000 word) phase 1 report, based largely on the site visits, will assess the match between today's health information systems and current plans for using electronic health records nationwide, identify important information management problems that could be solved relatively easily and inexpensively (i.e., where short payback periods and quick improvements would be possible) by today's technologies, provide (non-comprehensive) illustrations of how today's knowledge about computer science and IT could be used to provide immediate short-term benefits to the health care system, and lay out important questions that future reports (from this or other studies) should address.

In phase 2, the committee will prepare a phase 2 report identifying technical areas where additional computer science and IT research is needed to further advance the state of the art of health care IT; priorities for research that will yield significantly increased medical effectiveness or reduced costs; information management problems whose solutions require new practices and policies; and public policy questions that need to be resolved to allow such research to proceed.

Both reports are intended to identify technical solutions to advance health care IT, to expose the information technology and computer science research communities to important technical problems, and to provide a foundation for other studies related to health care informatics.

with a health and biomedical emphasis that is largely lacking in the world of computer science research. In the context of this report, specialists in health/biomedical informatics can serve a bridging function between the computer science community and the world of biomedicine with which computer science researchers are largely unfamiliar.

The committee thanks the National Library of Medicine, the National Institute of Biomedical Imaging and Bioengineering, the National Science Foundation, the Vanderbilt University Medical Center, Partners Health-Care System, the Robert Wood Johnson Foundation, and the Commonwealth Fund for the financial support needed to conduct this study.

For providing information and hosting site visits for the committee, the committee expresses its appreciation to a number of organizations: Partners HealthCare (David Bates, Henry Chueh, Anuj Dalal, John Glaser, and Jeff Schnipper), the University of Pittsburgh Medical Center (Jocelyn Benes, Jody Cervenak, Jacque Dailey, Steven Docimo, Tom

Dongilli, William Fera, Kim Gracey, Robert Kormos, James Levin, Daniel Martich, Ed McCallister, Tami Merryman, Sean O'Rourke, Vivek Reddy, Paul Sikora, Michele Steimer, and Jeff Szymanski), HCA Tristar (David Archer, Darryl Campbell, Kimberly Lewis, Annette Matlock, Jon Perlin, Melody Rose, Ruth Westcott, and Kelly Wood), Intermountain Healthcare (Lynn Elstein, Stan Huff, Marc Probst, and Brent Wallace), the Palo Alto Medical Foundation (Albert Chan, Steve Hansen, Neil Knutsen, Charlotte Mitchell, Tomas Moran, Gil Radtke, and Paul Tang), the University of California, San Francisco (Sharon Friend, Gail Harden, Michael Kamerick, Jon Showstack, and Deborah Yano-Fong), Vanderbilt University Medical Center (Rashid M. Ahmad, John Doulis, Mark Frisse, David Gregory, Ken Holroyd, Sara Hutchison, Marsha Kedigh, Randy Miller, Neal Patel, Corey Slovis, and Jack Starmer), San Francisco General Hospital (Geoff Manley), and the Department of Veterans Affairs (Stanlie Daniels, Neil Eldridge, Neil Evans, Ross Fletcher, Raya Kheirbek, Tracie Loving, Joaquin Martinez, Linwood Moore, Fernando O. Rivera, and Kenneth Steadman).

A number of individuals also briefed the committee during open sessions: B. Alton Brantley (principal, the CCI Group), Kenneth D. Mandl (Harvard Medical School and Harvard-MIT Division of Health Sciences and Technology), Greg Walton (HIMSS Analytics), Denis Cortese (Mayo Clinic), Peter Neupert (Microsoft), Scott Wallace (National Coalition for Health Care IT), Janet Corrigan (National Quality Forum), Alicia A. Bradford (Office of the National Coordinator for Health Information Technology), Peter J. Fabri (University of South Florida and Northwestern University), and Gina Grumke and Monique Lambert (Intel). Betsy Humphreys and Donald A.B. Lindberg from the National Library of Medicine provided the charge to the committee at its first meeting.

The committee also appreciates the efforts of David Padgham, associate program officer, who left the National Research Council in May 2008, in organizing these site visits and other information-gathering sessions of the committee. Finally, the committee thanks Herbert Lin, study director and chief scientist of the Computer Science and Telecommunications Board, for his counsel throughout the project and his effort in developing the report.

Acknowledgment of Reviewers

This report has been reviewed in draft form by individuals chosen for their diverse perspectives and technical expertise, in accordance with procedures approved by the National Research Council's Report Review Committee. The purpose of this independent review is to provide candid and critical comments that will assist the institution in making its published report as sound as possible and to ensure that the report meets institutional standards for objectivity, evidence, and responsiveness to the study charge. The review comments and draft manuscript remain confidential to protect the integrity of the deliberative process. We wish to thank the following individuals for their review of this report:

Gregory D. Abowd, Georgia Institute of Technology,
Alton Brantley, Cardinal Consulting, Inc.,
Janet Corrigan, National Quality Forum,
Peter J. Fabri, University of South Florida College of Medicine,
Chuck Geschke, Adobe Systems,
Sara Kiesler, Carnegie Mellon University,
Isaac Kohane, Harvard University,
Prasenjit Mitra, Pennsylvania State University,
Peter Neupert, Microsoft Corporation,
Ted Shortliffe, University of Arizona College of Medicine, Phoenix, and
Lee Sproull, New York University.

Although the reviewers listed above have provided many constructive comments and suggestions, they were not asked to endorse the conclusions or recommendations, nor did they see the final draft of the report before its release. The review of this report was overseen by David G. Hoel of the Medical University of South Carolina and Victor Vyssotsky. Appointed by the National Research Council, they were responsible for making certain that an independent examination of this report was carried out in accordance with institutional procedures and that all review comments were carefully considered. Responsibility for the final content of this report rests entirely with the authoring committee and the institution.

Contents

SUMMARY   1

1   HEALTH CARE IN THE UNITED STATES TODAY   13
    1.1 The Tasks and Workflow of Health Care, 14
    1.2 The Institution and Economics of Health Care, 15
    1.3 Current Implementations of Health Care Information
         Technology, 17
    1.4 Trends, 17
    1.5 The Structure of This Report, 18

2   A VISION FOR 21st CENTURY HEALTH CARE   19
    AND WELLNESS

3   CROSSING THE HEALTH CARE IT CHASM   25

4   PRINCIPLES FOR SUCCESS   30
    4.1 Evolutionary Change, 31
         4.1.1 Principle 1: Focus on Improvements in Care—
                Technology Is Secondary, 31
         4.1.2 Principle 2: Seek Incremental Gain from Incremental
                Effort, 32
         4.1.3 Principle 3: Record Available Data So That They Can Be
                Used for Care, Process Improvement, and Research, 32

4.1.4 Principle 4: Design for Human and Organization Factors, 32

4.1.5 Principle 5: Support the Cognitive Functions of All Caregivers, Including Health Professionals, Patients, and Their Families, 33

4.2 Radical Change, 33

4.2.1 Principle 6: Architect Information and Workflow Systems to Accommodate Disruptive Change, 33

4.2.2 Principle 7: Archive Data for Subsequent Re-interpretation, 34

4.2.3 Principle 8: Seek and Develop Technologies That Identify and Eliminate Ineffective Work Processes, 34

4.2.4 Principle 9: Seek and Develop Technologies That Clarify the Context of Data, 35

5 RESEARCH CHALLENGES   36

5.1 An Overarching Research Grand Challenge: Patient-Centered Cognitive Support, 39

5.2 Other Representative Research Challenges, 45

5.2.1 Modeling, 45

5.2.2 Automation, 46

5.2.3 Data Sharing and Collaboration, 49

5.2.4 Data Management at Scale, 53

5.2.5 Automated Full Capture of Physician-Patient Interactions, 56

6 RECOMMENDATIONS   59

6.1 Government, 60

6.2 The Computer Science Community, 65

6.3 Health Care Organizations, 66

7 CONCLUDING THOUGHTS   68

APPENDIXES

A Committee Members and Staff   71
B Meeting and Site Visit Agendas and Site Visit Methodology   80
C Observations, Consequences, and Opportunities: The Site Visits of the Committee   93

Summary

BACKGROUND AND INTRODUCTION

Health care is an information- and knowledge-intensive enterprise. In the future, health care providers will need to rely increasingly on information technology (IT) to acquire, manage, analyze, and disseminate health care information and knowledge. Many studies have identified deficiencies in the current health care system, including inadequate care, superfluous or incorrect care, immense inefficiencies and hence high costs, and inequities in access to care. In response, federal policy makers have tended to focus on the creation and interchange of electronic health information and the use of IT as critical infrastructural improvements whose deployments help to address some (but by no means all) of these deficiencies.

Any systematic effort to change the medical and health information management paradigm from one based on paper to one based on IT must address two basic challenges: using the best technology available today to build and deploy systems in the short term and identifying the gaps between the best of today's technology and what is ultimately needed to improve health care. The first provides opportunities for near-term improvement; the second informs basic research and the design of future systems.

The present study was chartered by its sponsors to help elucidate how the computer science research community can help to meet both of these challenges. Members of this community are familiar with the newest ideas in computer science and are thus in a position both to offer insight into how they might apply to the health care problems of today and to identify opportunities for new advances. However, the study described in this report was conducted by an interdisciplinary committee of experts not only from the computer science community (including members with expertise in fields such as databases, security, networking, human-computer interaction, and large-scale system deployments), but also from health/biomedical informatics and from health care per se (e.g., physicians who have worked with information technologies) to provide a suitable grounding in the realities of and thinking in these disciplines.

By design, the effort of the Committee on Engaging the Computer Science Research Community in Health Care Informatics was both time- and resource-limited. In its work, the committee focused primarily on understanding the nature and impact of the IT investments made by major health care organizations. Thus, this study does not touch except in the most peripheral way on a myriad of complex social, political, and economic issues that complicate the task of health care reform.

The evidentiary basis for this study involves several threads. The primary observational evidence was derived from committee site visits to eight medical centers around the country—for the most part acknowledged leaders in applying IT to health care—on the theory that many of the important innovations and achievements for health care IT would be found in such organizations thought to be leaders in the field. In addition, this study built on previous work of the Institute of Medicine (IOM) and the National Academy of Engineering on health care (specifically, the committee adopted as a point of departure the IOM series "Crossing the Quality Chasm"[1]) and on a selective literature review.

These multiple sources of evidence—viewed from the committee's perspective—suggest that current efforts aimed at the nationwide deployment of health care IT will not be sufficient to achieve the vision of 21st century health care, and may even set back the cause if these efforts continue wholly without change from their present course. Specifically, success in this regard will require greater emphasis on providing cognitive support for health care providers and for patients and family caregivers on the part of computer science and health/biomedical informatics researchers. Vendors, health care organizations, and government will also have to pay attention to cognitive support, which refers to computer-based tools and systems that offer clinicians and patients assistance for thinking about and solving problems related to specific instances of health care. This point is the central conclusion of this report.

---

[1]Institute of Medicine, *Crossing the Quality Chasm: A New Health System for the 21st Century*, The National Academies Press, Washington, D.C., 2005, available at http://www.nap.edu/catalog.php?record_id=10027.

HEALTH CARE IN THE UNITED STATES TODAY

It is widely recognized that today's health care fails to deliver the most effective care and suffers substantially as a result of medical errors. In addition, many medical interventions undertaken today are in fact not necessary. These persistent problems do not reflect incompetence on the part of health care professionals—rather, they are a consequence of the inherent intellectual complexity of health care taken as a whole and a medical care environment that has not been adequately structured to help clinicians avoid mistakes or to systematically improve their decision making and practice. Administrative and organizational fragmentation, together with complex, distributed, and unclear authority and responsibility, further complicates the health care environment.

Many of the relevant factors can be classified largely into three distinct areas: the tasks and workflow of health care, the institution and economics of health care, and the nature of health care IT as it is currently implemented.

- *The tasks and workflow of health care.* Health care decisions often require reasoning under high degrees of uncertainty about a patient's medical state and the effectiveness of past and future treatments for the particular patient. In addition, medical workflows are often complex and non-transparent and are characterized by many interruptions, inadequately defined roles and responsibilities, poorly kept and managed schedules, and little documentation of steps, expectations, and outcomes. Complex care is increasingly provided to patients in a time- and resource-pressured environment because of the need to contain costs.
- *The institution and economics of health care.* The large number of health care payers and coverage plans, each with its own rules for coverage, complicates administration. In addition, incentives for payment are often distorted or perverse, leading (for example) to more generous compensation for medical procedures than for communication with patients or for diagnosis or preventive care. Patients and providers must also navigate a confusing landscape of tertiary care centers, community hospitals, clinics, primary and specialist doctors and other providers, payers, health plans, and information sources.
- *Current implementations of health care IT.* Many health care organizations do spend considerable money on IT, but the IT is often implemented in systems in a monolithic fashion that makes even small changes hard to introduce. Furthermore, IT applications appear designed largely to automate tasks or business processes. They are often designed in ways that simply mimic existing paper-based forms and provide little support for the cognitive tasks of clinicians or the workflow of the people who must actually use the system. Moreover, these applications do not take advan-

tage of human-computer interaction principles, leading to poor designs that can increase the chance of error, add to rather than reduce work, and compound the frustrations of executing required tasks. As a result, these applications sometimes increase workload, and they can introduce new forms of error that are difficult to detect.

A number of trends will put additional pressure for change on the health care environment. These trends include an aging population and a corresponding increase in the complexity and weight of the disease burden, the emergence of genome-based personalized medicine, a larger role for patients in managing their own health care, and yet greater emphasis on efficiency and cost control in health care. As a result, health care processes will become more complex and more time-constrained, and the demands placed on care providers will become more intense.

A VISION FOR 21st CENTURY HEALTH CARE AND WELLNESS

The IOM defines health care quality as "the degree to which health services for individuals and populations increase the likelihood of desired health outcomes and are consistent with current professional knowledge,"[2] and in recent years, a broad consensus has emerged on the future health care environment. In the words of the IOM, health care should be safe, effective, patient-centered, timely, efficient, and equitable.[3] Achieving this vision entails many different factors (e.g., systemic changes in how to pay for health care, an emphasis on disease prevention rather than disease treatment), but none is more important than the effective use of information.

The committee identified seven information-intensive aspects of the IOM's vision for 21st century health care:

• Comprehensive data on patients' conditions, treatments, and outcomes;
• Cognitive support for health care professionals and patients to help integrate patient-specific data where possible and account for any uncertainties that remain;
• Cognitive support for health care professionals to help integrate evidence-based practice guidelines and research results into daily practice;

---

[2]Institute of Medicine, *Medicare: A Strategy for Quality Assurance*, National Academy Press, Washington, D.C., 1990, available at http://www.nap.edu/catalog.php?record_id=1547.

[3]Institute of Medicine, *Crossing the Quality Chasm: A New Health System for the 21st Century*, The National Academies Press, Washington, D.C., 2005, available at http://www.nap.edu/catalog.php?record_id=10027.

- Instruments and tools that allow clinicians to manage a portfolio of patients and to highlight problems as they arise both for an individual patient and within populations;
- Rapid integration of new instrumentation, biological knowledge, treatment modalities, and so on into a "learning" health care system that encourages early adoption of promising methods but also analyzes all patient experience as experimental data;
- Accommodation of growing heterogeneity of locales for provision of care, including home instrumentation for monitoring and treatment, lifestyle integration, and remote assistance; and
- Empowerment of patients and their families in effective management of health care decisions and their implementation, including personal health records, education about the individual's conditions and options, and support of timely and focused communication with professional health care providers.

CROSSING THE HEALTH CARE IT CHASM

The committee observed a number of success stories in the implementation of health care IT. But although seeing these successes was encouraging, they fall far short, even in the aggregate, of what is needed to support the IOM's vision of quality health care. IT-related activities of health professionals observed by the committee in these organizations were rarely well integrated into clinical practice. Health care IT was rarely used to provide clinicians with evidence-based decision support and feedback; to support data-driven process improvement; or to link clinical care and research. Health care IT rarely provided an integrative view of patient data. Care providers spent a great deal of time in electronically documenting what they did for patients, but these providers often said that they were entering the information to comply with regulations or to defend against lawsuits, rather than because they expected someone to use it to improve clinical care. Health care IT implementation time lines were often measured in decades, and most systems were poorly or incompletely integrated into practice.

Although the use of health care IT is an integral element of health care in the 21st century, the current focus of the health care IT efforts that the committee observed is not sufficient to drive the kind of change in health care that is truly needed. The nation faces a health care IT chasm that is analogous to the quality chasm highlighted by the IOM over the past decade. So that the nation can cross the health care IT chasm, the committee advocates re-balancing the portfolio of investments in health care IT to place a greater emphasis on providing cognitive support for health care providers, patients, and family caregivers; observing proven principles for success in designing and implementing IT; and accelerating research related to health care in the computer and social sciences and in health/biomedical informatics.

PRINCIPLES FOR SUCCESS

Change in the health care system can be viewed from two equally important perspectives—those of evolutionary and of radical change. Evolutionary change means continuous, iterative improvement of existing processes sustained over long periods of time. Radical change means qualitatively new ways of conceptualizing and solving health and health care problems and revolutionary ways of addressing those problems. Any approach to health care IT should enable and anticipate both types of change since they work together over time.

The committee identified five principles related to evolutionary change and four related to radical change to guide successful use of health care IT to support a 21st century vision of health care. These principles are elaborated in Chapter 4.

Principles for Evolutionary Change

1. Focus on improvements in care—technology is secondary.
2. Seek incremental gain from incremental effort.
3. Record available data so that today's biomedical knowledge can be used to interpret the data to drive care, process improvement, and research.
4. Design for human and organizational factors so that social and institutional processes will not pose barriers to appropriately taking advantage of technology.
5. Support the cognitive functions of all caregivers, including health professionals, patients, and their families.

Principles for Radical Change

6. Architect information and workflow systems to accommodate disruptive change.
7. Archive data for subsequent re-interpretation, that is, in anticipation of future advances in biomedical knowledge that may change today's interpretation of data and advances in computer science that may provide new ways of extracting meaningful and useful knowledge from existing data stores.
8. Seek and develop technologies that identify and eliminate ineffective work processes.
9. Seek and develop technologies that clarify the context of data.

RESEARCH CHALLENGES

There are deep intellectual research challenges at the nexus of health care and computer science (and health/biomedical informatics as well). The committee found it useful to conceptualize necessary research efforts along two separate dimensions. The first dimension is the extent to which new fundamental, general-purpose research is needed. Some problems in health care can be seen as having solutions on a relatively clear path forward from existing technologies (e.g., aggregation of patient health care information into a common data repository), whereas others are genuinely advanced problems (e.g., aggregation of patient health care information into a trustworthy database with explicit representation of uncertainty). (Also, note that this first dimension aligns to a large degree with the evolutionary/radical change dichotomy described above, where evolutionary change can be associated with straightforward extrapolation of current knowledge and technology, and radical change with problem domains that will require successes in fundamental research.)

A second dimension is the extent to which new research specific to health care and biomedicine is needed. This second dimension is rooted in the observation that some advances needed for improving health care are general problems in computer science (e.g., achieving high availability with low system management overhead), and others are highly specific to health care (e.g., developing high-quality devices for human-computer interaction that do not inadvertently help to spread infection as care providers move from patient to patient). This distinction is helpful because a broad coalition might fund and pursue the former, whereas the latter might be of interest to a narrower set in the health and biomedical informatics communities.

During the committee's discussions, patient-centered cognitive support emerged as an overarching grand research challenge to focus health-related efforts of the computer science research community, which can play an important role in helping to cross the health care IT chasm.

An Overarching Research Grand Challenge:
Patient-Centered Cognitive Support

Much of health care is transactional—admitting a patient, encountering a patient at the bedside or clinic, ordering a drug, interpreting a report, or handing off a patient. Yet transactions are only the operational expression of an understanding of the patient and a set of goals and plans for that patient. Clinicians have in mind a conceptual model of the patient reflecting their understanding of interacting physiological, psychological, societal, and other dimensions. They use new findings—raw data—to refine their understanding of the model they are using. Then, based on medical knowledge, medical logic, and mostly heuristic decision making, they make orders (transactions) that they hope will improve the condition of or even cure the (real) patient.

Today, clinicians spend a great deal of time and energy searching and sifting through raw data about patients and trying to integrate these data with their general medical knowledge to form relevant mental abstractions and associations relevant to the patient's situation. Such sifting efforts force clinicians to devote precious cognitive resources to the details of data and make it more likely that they will overlook some important higher-order consideration.

The health care IT systems of today tend to squeeze all cognitive support for the clinician through the lens of health care transactions and the related raw data, without an underlying representation of a conceptual model for the patient showing how data fit together and which are important or unimportant. As a result, an understanding of the patient can be lost amidst all the data, all the tests, and all the monitoring equipment.

In the committee's vision of patient-centered cognitive support, the clinician interacts with models and abstractions of the patient that place the raw data into context and synthesize them with medical knowledge in ways that make clinical sense for that patient. Raw data are still available, but they are not the direct focus of the clinician. These virtual patient models are the computational counterparts of the clinician's conceptual model of a patient. They depict and simulate a theory about interactions going on in the patient and enable patient-specific parameterization and multicomponent alerts. They build on submodels of biological and physiological systems and also of epidemiology that take into account, for example, the local prevalence of diseases. The use of these models to establish clinical context would free the clinician from having to make direct sense of raw data, and thus he or she would have a much easier time defining, testing, and exploring his/her own working theory. What links the raw data to the abstract models might be called medical logic—that is, computer-based tools that examine raw data relevant to a specific patient and suggest their clinical implications given the context of the models and abstractions. Computers can then provide decision support—that is, tools that help clinicians decide on a course of action in response to an understanding of the patient's status. At the same time, although clinicians can work with abstractions that keep them from being overwhelmed by data, they must also have the ability to access the raw data as needed if they wish to explore the presented interpretations and abstractions in greater depth.

There are many challenging computer science research problems associated with this vision. Future clinician and patient-facing systems would draw on the data, information, and knowledge obtained in both patient care and research to provide decision support sensitive to work-flow and human factors. The decision support systems would explicitly incorporate patient utilities, values, and resource constraints (e.g., cost-effectiveness analysis, value of information, and so on). They would support holistic plans, intentions, and multiple decision makers. They would allow users to simulate interventions on the virtual patient before doing them for real. These decision support systems would have transactions built into them to help users carry out orders, in contrast to today's systems in which decision support is commonly an add-on to systems and is designed primarily for transaction processing. Rather than having data entered by clinicians into computer systems, the content of clinical inter-actions would be captured in self-documenting environments with little or no additional effort on the part of the clinicians. (That is, an intelligent, sensor-rich environment would monitor clinical interactions and reduce sensor input to notes that document the medically significant content of those interactions.)

In addition to the research challenges related to modeling the virtual patient and biomedical knowledge, there are challenges in modeling and supporting multiplayer decision making (e.g., involving family, patient, primary care provider, specialist, payer, and so on). Techniques to inter-connect the components are likely to be equally challenging.

Other Representative Research Challenges

• *Modeling.* One aspect of the virtual patient involves modeling vari-ous subsystems within a real patient (e.g., different organs, digestive system, and so on) to show how they interact. One approach to modeling physiological subsystems in a specific patient is to appropriately param-eterize a generic model of those subsystems. But finding appropriate parameterizations for any given model and coupling the different models and the data to drive them pose significant intellectual challenges. For example, coupling models will require a computational platform that can support multiple interacting components that can be combined into larger and more complex models. Such a platform must not only support parallel operation of the analytical processes but also allow assembly of hierarchical simulation and information structures, dynamically built, exploited, modified when possible on the basis of empirical data, and abandoned when no longer effective.

• *Automation.* When automated systems are deployed in an opera-tional environment, they must work harmoniously with each other. But in practice, because they have been developed in isolation, they do not, with the result that they provide contradictory signaling and have dif-ferent monitoring requirements and raise different safety concerns. Most importantly, they raise issues of trust in these systems—excessive trust leads personnel to believe erroneous indicators and operations, while inadequate trust forces them to check up on these systems, wasting valuable time. Overcoming these operational integration problems for automated systems remains a major challenge.

• *Data sharing and collaboration.* The data relevant to health care are highly heterogeneous. To exploit such data effectively, users need to be able to ask queries that span multiple data sources without requiring the data to be standardized or requiring the user to query each single database in isolation. Today, data integration usually entails a major and costly effort. Research challenges in this area involve data integration systems that are fundamentally easier to use, data integration methodologies that can proceed incrementally while remaining compatible with previous versions, and more flexible architectures for data sharing and integration.

• *Data management at scale.* Presuming the existence of large integrated corpora of data, another major challenge is in managing those data. Some of the important dimensions of medical information management include annotation and metadata, linkage, and privacy.

• *Automated full capture of physician-patient interactions.* Such capture would release clinician time for more productive uses and help to ensure more complete and timely patient records. Some of the important dimensions in this problem domain include real-time transcription and interpretation of the dialog between patient and provider, summarization of physical interactions between patient and provider based on the interpretation of images recorded by various cameras in the patient care room (subject to appropriate privacy safeguards), and correlation of the information contained in the audio and visual transcripts.

RECOMMENDATIONS

Government

Federal and state governments play important roles as supporters of research, payers for health care, and stimulators for education. The committee believes that government organizations—especially the federal government—should explicitly embrace measurable health care quality improvement as the driving rationale for its health care IT adoption efforts, and should shun programs that focus on promoting the adoption of specific clinical applications. Although this principle should not be taken to discourage incentives to invest in infrastructure (networks, workstations, administrative transaction processing systems, platforms for data mining, data repositories, and so on) that provides a foundation on which other specific clinical applications can be built, a top-down focus on specific clinical applications is likely to result in a premature "freezing" of inefficient workflows and processes and to impede iterative change.

In focusing on the goal to be achieved, namely better and/or less expensive health care, clinicians and other providers will appropriately be drawn to IT only if, where, and when it can be shown to enable them to do their jobs more effectively. Blanket promotion of IT adoption where benefits are not clear or are oversold—especially in a non-infrastructure context—will only waste resources and sour clinicians on the true potential of health care IT.

IT can be a fundamental enabler for both large-scale and small-scale improvement efforts. Because many health care groups have capacities for only a few large-scale improvement methods at a time, small-scale optimization is an important complement. An example of a small-scale optimization would be the use of a guideline alert system that enables individual physicians and/or their clinical teams to continually target areas of practice for self-improvement on guideline-concordant care. But for the most part, the health care IT available in today's market is not well suited to support small-scale optimization, which requires applications that are rapidly customizable in the field by end users. Federally inspired or supported initiatives that incentivize health care organizations to achieve iterative small-scale optimization and subsequent translation of successes to a larger scale are likely to help stimulate the creation of a new market for these customizable applications.

This analysis leads to six important recommendations for the federal government:

- Incentivize clinical performance gains rather than acquisition of IT per se.
- Encourage initiatives to empower iterative process improvement and small-scale optimization.
- Encourage development of standards and measures of health care IT performance related to cognitive support for health professionals and patients, adaptability to support iterative process improvement, and effective use to improve quality.
- Encourage interdisciplinary research in three critical areas: (a) organizational systems-level research into the design of health care systems, processes, and workflow; (b) computable knowledge structures and models for medicine needed to make sense of available patient data including preferences, health behaviors, and so on; and (c) human-computer interaction in a clinical context.
- Encourage (or at least do not impede) efforts by health care organizations and communities to aggregate data about health care people,

processes, and outcomes from all sources subject to appropriate protection of privacy and confidentiality.

• Support additional education and training efforts at the intersection of health care, computer science, and health/biomedical informatics. Current programs of the National Library of Medicine and other institutes of the National Institutes of Health are exemplars of such support.

The Computer Science Community

The computer science community can find deep, meaningful, and fundamental intellectual challenges in the health care problem domain (as indicated above). Accordingly, the committee believes that the computer science community should:

• Engage as co-equal intellectual partners and collaborators with health care practitioners and experts in health/biomedical informatics and other relevant disciplines, such as industrial and process engineering and design, in an ongoing relationship to understand and solve problems of importance to health care.

• Develop institutional mechanisms within academia for rewarding work at the health care/computer science interface.

• Support educational and retraining efforts for computer science researchers who want to explore research opportunities in health care.

Health Care Organizations

The senior management in health care organizations and health care payers have often taken the lead in the deployment of IT for health care. They should:

• Organize incentives, roles, workflow, processes, and supporting infrastructure to encourage, support, and respond to opportunities for clinical performance gains.

• Balance the institution's IT portfolio among automation, connectivity, decision support, and data-mining capabilities.

• Develop the necessary data infrastructure for health care improvement by aggregating data regarding people, processes, and outcomes from all sources.

• Insist that vendors supply IT that permits the separation of data from applications and facilitates data transfers to and from other non-vendor applications in shareble and generally useful formats.

• Seek IT solutions that yield incremental gains from incremental efforts.

1

Health Care in the United States Today

Today's health care fails to deliver the most cost-effective care and suffers substantially from medical errors and waste. One often-cited data point is the 1998 Institute of Medicine (IOM) estimate that preventable medical errors lead to as many as 98,000 deaths per year in the United States;[1] a more recent paper from 2005 suggests that there is still much more work to be done to make significant progress in reducing this figure.[2] It has been estimated that, on average, Americans receive about half of the medical care that is recommended for them.[3] Conversely, the available evidence suggests that many medical interventions undertaken today are in fact not necessary or are recommended without adequate personalization.[4] For example, based on an analysis of regional disparities in Medicare expenditures, Fisher et al. suggest that the United States as a whole could save annually up to 30 percent of Medicare expenditures

[1]Institute of Medicine, *To Err Is Human: Building a Safer Health System*, National Academy Press, Washington, D.C., 2000, available at http://www.nap.edu/catalog.php?record_id =9728.

[2]Lucian L. Leape and Donald M. Berwick, "Five Years After *To Err Is Human*: What Have We Learned?," *Journal of the American Medical Association* 293(19):2384-2390, 2005.

[3]Elizabeth A. McGlynn et al., "The Quality of Health Care Delivered to Adults in the United States," *New England Journal of Medicine* 348(26):2635-2645, 2003, available at http://content.nejm.org/cgi/content/abstract/348/26/2635.

[4]K.A. Kuhn et al., "Informatics and Medicine, from Molecules to Populations," *Methods of Information in Medicine* 47(4):296-317, 2008.

with no compromise in medical outcomes or patient satisfaction;[5] if so, resources might be freed to implement additional coverage for the uninsured and/or additional best practices that are not reflected in today's health care practices.

For the most part, these persistent problems do not reflect incompetence on the part of health care workers.[6] Instead, they are a consequence of the inherent intellectual complexity of health care taken as a whole and a medical care environment that provides insufficient help for clinicians to avoid mistakes or to inform their decision making and practice. Administrative and organizational fragmentation, together with complex, distributed, and unclear authority and responsibility, further complicates the health care environment.

Many of the relevant factors can be classified into three distinct areas: the tasks and workflow of health care, the institution and economics of health care, and the nature of health care IT as it is currently implemented. (In this report, observations from site visits are cross-referenced where appropriate with the notation CxOy. Cx refers to the Category x (1-6) of observation made in Table C.1 (Appendix C), and Oy refers by number (1-25) to a particular observation as listed in Table C.1.

1.1 THE TASKS AND WORKFLOW OF HEALTH CARE

• *Health care decisions that require reasoning in the face of uncertainty.* Sources of uncertainty include biological variability,[7] uncertainty about the medications that a patient is actually taking because of missing medical records at the point of care,[8] uncertainty about the effectiveness of past and future treatments for the particular patient [C1O1], simple randomness arising from inherently stochastic processes, and imperfect models or understanding of causality.

• *Complex and non-transparent workflow* [C2O6] that is characterized by many interruptions [C2O7], inadequately defined roles and responsibilities, poorly kept and managed schedules, and little documentation of

---

[5]Elliott S. Fisher et al., "The Implications of Regional Variations in Medicare Spending. Part 2: Health Outcomes and Satisfaction with Care," *Annals of Internal Medicine* 138(4):288-298, February 18, 2003.

[6]U.S. Department of Health and Human Services Factsheet: "Improving Patient Safety and Preventing Medical Errors," *HHS Factsheet*, March 25, 2002.

[7]Ute Schwarz et al., "Genetic Determinants of Response to Warfarin During Initial Anticoagulation," *New England Journal of Medicine* 358(10):999-1008, March 6, 2008.

[8]As much as 30 percent of the information an internist needs is often not accessible during a patient's visit because of missing clinical information and missing laboratory reports. See D.G. Covell, G.C. Uman, and P.R. Manning, "Information Needs in Office Practice: Are They Being Met?," *Annals of Internal Medicine* 103(4):596-599, 1995.

steps, expectations, and outcomes.[9] Poor information flow is particularly apparent at the interfaces of health care (e.g., when a patient transitions from inpatient to outpatient, when nurses change shifts) [C2O5].

• *Increasing complexity of the care provided to patients in a time-pressured environment.*[10] The aging patient population has a growing number of chronic disease conditions that must be managed.[11] According to Yarnall et al.,[12] managing in accordance with the preventive guidelines relevant to "average" adult patients would require an average of approximately 40 minutes per patient per year. A typical patient sees his primary care physician only 4 times a year for a 15-minute appointment (for a total of 60 minutes of interaction), which would leave only 20 minutes per year (60 minutes − 40 minutes) for everything other than matters related to the guidelines for preventive care (by 2030, about half of all Americans will have at least one chronic disease).[13]

1.2 THE INSTITUTION AND ECONOMICS OF HEALTH CARE

• *A large number of payers for health care, each with their own rules for coverage.* For example, a large medical center may have to handle the complexity associated with managing thousands of different health insurance plans.[14] A typical family physician or internist in the United States wastes

---

[9]See, for example, S. Panzarasa et al., "Improving Compliance to Guidelines Through Workflow Technology: Implementation and Results in a Stroke Unit," *Studies in Health Technology and Informatics* 129(Pt. 2):834-839, 2007.

[10]Center for Studying Health System Change. Physician Survey, available at http://CTSonline.s-3.com/psurvey.asp.

[11]Brian Raymond and Cynthia Dold, *Clinical Information Systems: Achieving the Vision*, Kaiser Permanente Institute for Health Policy, Oakland, Calif., February 2002, available at http://www.kpihp.org/publications/docs/clinical_information.pdf.

[12]Kimberly S.H. Yarnall, Kathryn I. Pollak, Truls Østbye, Katrina M. Krause, and J. Lloyd Michener, "Primary Care: Is There Enough Time for Prevention?," *American Journal of Public Health* 93(4):635-641, April 2003, available at http://www.ajph.org/cgi/content/full/93/4/635.

[13]Shin-Yi Wu and Anthony Green, *Projection of Chronic Illness Prevalence and Cost Inflation*, RAND Corporation, October 2000.

[14]Respondents to an informal poll of the ACMI discussion list in June 2008 indicated that their home organizations (medical centers) often had to cope with many dozens of health care payers (usually insurers), each of which had hundreds of different plans with different rules for coverage. (ACMI, the American College of Medical Informatics, consists of elected fellows from the United States and abroad who have made significant and sustained contributions to the field of medical informatics.) The range reported was from a low of 578 plans to a high in excess of 20,000.

40 to 50 minutes each day on dealing with managed care administrative hassles.[15]

• *Distorted or perverse incentives for payment.* For example, as a general rule, health care providers are compensated more readily and more generously for performing medical procedures than for communication and cognitive work such as diagnosis or preventive care. In many cases, the reimbursement rate is higher when patients develop complications rather than when patients receive quality care—that is, physicians are generally paid to fix the problems their medical care may have caused or did not prevent.[16] In addition, the current medical care system offers little recognition or reward for coordinating care and pays primarily for face-to-face (office) visits.[17]

• *A fragmented and "siloed" environment of health care organizations.* Both patients and providers must navigate a confusing landscape of tertiary care centers, community hospitals, clinics, primary and specialist doctors and other providers, payers, health plans, and information sources.[18]

• *Increasing tightness in the health care labor market for certain specialties,* such as nurses,[19] primary care physicians,[20] health care paraprofessionals, and clinicians with informatics training. (Health/biomedical informatics training is not generally a requirement in most curricula for health care professionals, thus contributing to a scarcity of individuals so trained.)

---

[15]L.S. Sommers, T.W. Hacker, D.M. Schneider, P.A. Pugno, and J.B. Garrett, "A Descriptive Study of Managed Care Hassles in 26 Practices," *Western Journal of Medicine* 174(3):175-179, 2001. The term "hassles" was used in the study to refer to issues that interject themselves directly into the doctor-patient visit, including "restricted formularies, limited access to medical specialists, the requirement of prior approvals for procedures, unavailable treatments, lengthy appeals processes, and physician payment delays."

[16]Vinod K. Sahney, "Engineering and the Health Care Organization," in National Academy of Engineering and Institute of Medicine, *Building a Better Delivery System: A New Engineering/Health Care Partnership*, The National Academies Press, Washington, D.C., 2005.

[17]Institute of Medicine, *Crossing the Quality Chasm: A New Health System for the 21st Century*, National Academy Press, Washington, D.C., March 2001. As a concrete example, the committee heard of the incentives for an insurance company to do very little for a 62-year-old man developing type 2 diabetes because the costly complications would most likely arise after he turns 65, and would thus be covered by Medicare. Pay-for-performance programs are a notable exception to such perverse incentives, although they have not been widely adopted.

[18]Thomas Bodenheimer, "Coordinating Care—A Perilous Journey Through the Health Care System," *New England Journal of Medicine* 358(10):1064-1071, March 6, 2008.

[19]D.E. Hecker, "Occupational Employment Projections to 2014," *Monthly Labor Review* 128(11):70-101, 2005.

[20]National Association of Community Health Centers, "Access Transformed: Building a Primary Care Workforce for the 21st Century," Washington, D.C., 2008, available at http://www.nachc.com/client/documents/ACCESS%20Transformed%20full%20report.PDF.

1.3 CURRENT IMPLEMENTATIONS OF HEALTH CARE INFORMATION TECHNOLOGY

• *Monolithic and "siloed" information technology.* Many health care organizations, especially large ones, do spend considerable money on information technology (IT), but the IT is implemented in ways that make even small improvements hard to introduce [C4O14]. Even across the systems within an organization, interoperability is often awkward and slow [C4O14, C5O21, C5O23]. Information exchange with the information systems of other organizations is rare.[21]

• *IT applications that appear designed to automate tasks or business processes for administrative efficiency,[22] and that provide little support for the cognitive tasks of clinicians* [C1O4 and confirmed by IOM[23]]. IT-based systems for health care are often designed in ways that simply mimic existing paper-based forms and workflow [C1O2, C1O3] and do not take advantage of human-computer interaction principles [C5O20]. One result is poor system design that can increase the chance of error, add to rather than reduce workflow, and compound the frustrations of doing the required tasks. As a result, the computer system frequently increases the workload (for example, lack of trust in a system may force providers to maintain duplicate paper-based data records) and can introduce new forms of error that are difficult to detect. Complex policy and implementation issues relating to protecting privacy also make automation significantly more difficult.

1.4 TRENDS

A number of trends will put additional pressure for change on the health care environment. These trends include an aging population and a corresponding increase in the complexity and weight of the disease burden, the emergence of genome-based personalized medicine,[24] a larger

---

[21]J. Halamka, J.M. Overhage, L. Ricciardi, W. Rishel, C. Shirky, and C. Diamond, "Exchanging Health Information: Local Distribution, National Coordination," *Health Affairs* (Millwood) 24(5):1170-1179, 2005.

[22]William Stead, "Challenges in Informatics," in National Academy of Engineering and Institute of Medicine, *Building a Better Delivery System: A New Engineering/Health Care Partnership,* The National Academies Press, Washington, D.C., 2005.

[23]Institute of Medicine, *Building a Better Delivery System: A New Engineering/Health Care Partnership,* 2005, p. 15. See also Institute of Medicine, *Crossing the Quality Chasm: A New Health System for the 21st Century,* National Academy Press, Washington, D.C., 2001, p. 67.

[24]For example, a 2008 study suggests the personalization of drug regimens based on genetic profiles as an important step toward the ultimate goal of providing individualized treatment guided by genetic information. See Amy I. Lynch, Eric Boerwinkle, Barry R. Davis, et al., "Pharmacogenetic Association of the NPPA T2238C Genetic Variant with Cardiovascular Disease Outcomes in Patients with Hypertension," *Journal of the American Medical*

role for patients in managing their own health care,[25] and yet greater emphasis on efficiency and cost control in health care. As a result, health care processes will become more complex and more time-constrained, and the demands placed on care providers will become more intense.

1.5 THE STRUCTURE OF THIS REPORT

Chapter 2 reviews the IOM vision of 21st century health care and wellness as the appropriate point of departure for the committee's work. Chapter 3 describes a chasm between current efforts to deploy health care IT and what the committee believes is needed to achieve the IOM vision. Chapter 4 describes the committee's perspective on principles for developing and deploying successful health care IT, with success defined as progress toward the IOM vision. Chapter 5 describes some illustrative research challenges for the computer science community that emerge from the IOM vision. Chapter 6 presents the committee's recommendations, based on the results of its study, for government, for the computer science community, and for health care organizations.

Association 299(3):296-307, 2008. See also K.A. Kuhn et al., "Informatics and Medicine, from Molecules to Populations," *Methods of Information in Medicine* 47(4):296-317, 2008.

[25]Institute of Medicine, *Building a Better Delivery System: A New Engineering/Health Care Partnership*, 2005, p. 65.

2

A Vision for 21st Century Health Care and Wellness

The Institute of Medicine (IOM) defines health care quality as "the degree to which health services for individuals and populations increase the likelihood of desired health outcomes and are consistent with current professional knowledge," and in recent years, a broad consensus has emerged on the future health care environment. In the words of the IOM, health care should be:[1]

- *Safe*—avoiding injuries to patients from the care that is intended to help them.
- *Effective*—providing services based on scientific knowledge to all who could benefit and refraining from providing services to those not likely to benefit, avoiding underuse and overuse, respectively.
- *Patient-centered*—providing care that is respectful of and responsive to individual patient preferences, needs, and values and ensuring that patient values guide all clinical decisions.
- *Timely*—reducing waits and sometimes harmful delays for both those who receive and those who give care.
- Efficient—avoiding waste, including waste of equipment, supplies, ideas, and energy.
- *Equitable*—providing care that does not vary in quality because of

[1]Institute of Medicine, *Crossing the Quality Chasm: A New Health System for the 21st Century*, National Academy Press, Washington, D.C., March 2001.

personal characteristics such as gender, ethnicity, geographic location, and socioeconomic status.

The IOM vision calls for a health care system that is systematically organized and acculturated in ways that make it easy and rewarding for providers and patients to do the right thing, at the right time, in the right place, and in the right way. This vision entails many different factors (e.g., systemic changes in paying for health care, an emphasis on disease prevention rather than disease treatment). But none is more important than the effective use of information.[2]

Based on its observations and expertise, the committee identified a number of information-intensive aspects of the IOM's vision for 21st century health care. Each bullet phrase below summarizes one of these important health care IT capabilities, followed by an illustrative vignette of what might be possible. The vignettes (displayed in italic type) are not comprehensive (i.e., they do not cover all aspects of the capability).

• Comprehensive data on patients' conditions, treatments, and outcomes.

A clinician needs to know what medications an elderly, memory-challenged patient is taking. Recognizing the important difference between medications prescribed and medications taken, the clinician asks the patient to bring all of his pill containers, both prescription and over-the-counter, to the appointment. She asks the patient to place all of the containers on a surface table computer, which automatically identifies the medications in each of the containers and counts the number of pills remaining in each container. The pill containers also carry RFID [radio-frequency identification] tags, on which the initial fill-up quantities of the containers are stored. The table can read these tags, and thereby make an inference about what pills were actually taken and provide information about likely compliance with a particular medication regime.[3] Farther in the future, recognizing the differences in how

---

[2]Institute of Medicine, *The Computer-Based Patient Record: An Essential Technology for Health Care* (Revised Edition), National Academy Press, Washington, D.C., 1997, available at http://www.nap.edu/openbook.php?isbn=0309055326; Institute of Medicine, *Key Capabilities of an Electronic Health Record System: Letter Report*, The National Academies Press, Washington, D.C., 2003, available at http://www.nap.edu/catalog.php?record_id=10781; Institute of Medicine, *Patient Safety: Achieving a New Standard for Care*, The National Academies Press, Washington, D.C., 2004, available at http://www.nap.edu/openbook.php?isbn=0309090776.

[3]If purchase history were available to provide information on when the container was filled, inferences could be made about the frequency and timing of pill-taking, rather than only the total number of pills taken.

individuals absorb or clear medications from their bodies, a blood sample of the patient in question is analyzed with a mass spectrometer or other similar device, and the resulting spectrum identifies the actual level of all drugs in the patient's body. Combined with information from the smart table, a profile of the patient's compliance and pharmacokinetics for each drug is generated. The clinical significance of the smart medications table and the mass spectrometer is that together they help to reduce uncertainty by synthesizing different views into the patient's medication history.

• Cognitive support for health care professionals and patients to help integrate patient-specific data where possible and account for any uncertainties that remain.[4]

A primary care clinician needs to monitor a patient's heart condition. Cardiac information is provided to the clinician not in the form of tables of numbers or individual EKG plots, but rather as an overlay on a visual animated structural model of the patient's heart (not a generic heart) derived from various imaging modalities. The system displays the relevant functional information in summary form and provides an image of the heart in operation driven by all of the data that have been collected about the patient over time. Different time scales are available for display, and the clinician can display an animated image of the patient's heart in operation as the patient is resting or exerting himself (i.e., in near-real time), or track how the structure of the heart has changed over the last 2 years using time-lapse-like sequences. Functional histories are also available. Histories are instantly available in easy-to-read form, with different parameter histories presented on similar-looking charts normalized to z-scores and timescales, showing upper and lower "normal" and physiologic bounds.[5] The clinician also has the ability to drill down to any supporting piece of information that underlies the display. The clinical significance of an animated structural model is that it drastically reduces the cognitive effort needed for the clinician to visualize the heart functioning in this particular patient, freeing her to use those cognitive resources for other related tasks. The model also helps the patient to understand the medical situation at hand and assists both clinician and patient in determining an appropriate course of action.

---

[4]In this report, "cognitive support" refers to IT-based tools and systems that provide users (clinicians and patients) with the information, abstractions, and models needed to achieve the IOM's vision of health care quality.

[5]See, for example, Seth Powsner and Edward Tufte, "Graphical Summary of Patient Status," *The Lancet* 344(8919):386-389, August 6, 1994, available at http://www.stottlerhenke. com/projects/IPDRA2/info_resources/powsner_tufte_graphical_patient_summary.pdf.

• Cognitive support for health care professionals to help integrate evidence-based practice guidelines and research results into daily practice.

A primary care clinician has a number of patients with various heart conditions. In order to help stay current with recent literature, he subscribes to alerts from the medical literature and learns that a particular heart disease guideline has been updated to include a new drug that reportedly prevents a difficult and expensive complication. After comparing it to other guidelines that he believes to be trustworthy, he decides to incorporate this new guideline into his practice. By clicking on a link, the clinician can download the guideline to his system, which also searches for and constructs several potential action flowcharts to meet the guideline's goals, based on an internal computable model of clinic workflow and resources. He selects one and his disease management dashboards, order sets, and reminder systems are updated. (A dashboard is an easily viewed display that summarizes the health status of multiple patients.) The clinical significance of the literature alert system is that it enables the clinician to keep current and to systematically translate new knowledge into his practice while enabling the clinician and the patient to decide on the appropriate course of treatment.

• Instruments and tools that allow providers to manage a portfolio of patients and to highlight problems as they arise both within individual patients and within populations.

The computer of an outpatient care provider displays the summary health status (a "dashboard") of her 300 diabetic patients with color-codes and carefully designed graphical displays for clinical measures of the disease (blood sugar levels, A1C counts, and so on) that provide rapid assessment, at a glance, of the status of all patients: those who are managing illnesses successfully, those requiring intervention, and those who are marginal cases. When a diabetic patient visits her, the system reviews applicable guidelines, customizes an order set to the patient's state and insurance plan (e.g., picks the preferred drug from the drug class), and reminds the physician to discuss the selected drug with the patient. Feedback indicating success is provided when the provider sees that the display indicators of her patients show successful management. The clinical significance of a summary health status display is that it gives the provider prompt feedback about where her attention is most needed in time to take corrective action.

• Rapid integration of new instrumentation, biological knowledge, treatment modalities, and so on, into a "learning" health care system that encourages early adoption of promising methods but also analyzes all patient experience as experimental data.

> *A pediatrician in Los Angeles finds herself working with an ever grow-ing set of young patients with severe asthma. A group of them have added her to their Facebook page where they run a special widget that shows her when and where they did moderate or high physical activity outdoors. The application does not rely on self-reporting. Rather, the young people run an application on their mobile phones that uploads an SMS message containing their current location every 30 seconds to a private account where an application processes and summarizes loca-tion-activity data generated from accelerometers on their phones. The doctor has recently introduced a new feature whereby her patients use special Bluetooth-equipped inhalers that report via the mobile phone each time the inhaler is used. The website then displays when and where they used their Bluetooth-enabled inhalers. In addition to viewing trends over time, and patterns based on time of year and day of the week, she runs an application that relates her patients' activity to real-time pollution expo-sure models made available by the city. She uses the data to make a case to the city about other possible activity locations (e.g., different outdoor parks) and is soon going to enable her patients to sign up for automated customized alerts when they are overexerting themselves under hazard-ous environmental conditions. The clinical significance of an automated activity reporting and processing system is that it provides reliable data on what patients actually do (rather than what they say they do) in a form that is easy to understand, as well as additional detail to link to other data sources to clarify patterns, and delivery that is timely enough to support real-time feedback in time to change behavior.*

• Accommodation of the growing heterogeneity of locales for the provision of care, including home instrumentation for monitoring and treatment, lifestyle integration, and remote assistance.

> *A diabetic patient wears an active sensor that provides continuous blood-sugar readings. When these readings approach levels that indi-cate that actions need to be taken (e.g., taking an insulin shot, eating something), the sensor provides an indication to the patient. Acting with the patient's prior consent, if the patient fails to take the necessary action (as would be indicated by increasingly dangerous readings), the sensor communicates with a cell phone to place a call to an emergency caregiver. Along with the patient's vital signs and intake information (name, present location, and so on), the call also provides a summary of the relevant readings so that the caregiver can be dispatched to the site*

of the emergency and be prepared for what action should be taken. The clinical significance of an active sensor is that emergency intervention can be requested in the absence of patient action, and that the emergency response can be provided in advance with information that would otherwise have to be gathered immediately upon arrival.

• Empowerment of patients and their families in effective management of health care decisions and execution, including personal health records (as contrasted to medical records held by care providers), education about the individual's conditions and options, and support of timely and focused communication with professional health care providers.

The son of an elderly man hospitalized by a stroke needs to know about his father's medical condition. Rather than waiting for hours by his father's bedside to intercept a physician on rounds so that he can obtain authoritative information, he logs into a secure application that makes his father's electronic health record (EHR) available on the Internet. But since he is not a physician himself, he invokes a data interpretation application that examines the data in the EHR and provides in lay language a summary of the important aspects of a patient's medical condition, previously provided treatments, and treatment options under consideration. The application provides an interpretation (and the reasoning behind the interpretation) that is comparable to that which an experienced clinician could provide. The clinical significance of an automated EHR lay interpretation system is that the family can be kept in the decision-making loop, in a culturally sensitive way and on a more timely basis than is possible today, and potentially avoid delays often involved when families need time to make decisions—since they learn relevant facts sooner (perhaps even days sooner), they can start the process sooner. In addition to the data flowing from caregivers, the son can also enter information based on his knowledge of his father's present state and medical history, providing caregivers with another source of information, and empowering the son to have a greater role in his father's treatment.

3

Crossing the Health Care IT Chasm

The committee observed a number of success stories in implementation of health care information technology (IT). For example, one organization had implemented a pharmacy/medication administration system in what appeared to be an exemplary fashion. Making extensive use of robotics and bar coding of medication, patients, and providers, this organization had implemented procedures and practices that apparently reduced error rates in dispensing and administration significantly. Another organization had almost completely transitioned to electronic clinical ordering and documentation in both its inpatient and outpatient facilities. Another had made progress in using evidence-based medicine through clinician-customizable order sets to decrease the variability of care. Another had implemented effective data support for management of clinical process improvement and was able to support systematic decisions about where to focus organizational energy and attention.

Although seeing these successes was encouraging, in the committee's judgment they fall far short, even in the aggregate, of what is needed to support the Institute of Medicine's (IOM's) vision of quality health care. Apart from a few exceptional examples, the IT-related activities of health professionals observed by the committee in these organizations were not well integrated into clinical practice [C1O1, C1O2, C1O3, C4O17, C5O22, C6O24]. Health care IT was rarely used to provide clinicians with evidence-based decision support and feedback [C1O4]; to support data-driven process improvement [C2O6]; or to link clinical care and research [C2O10]. The committee saw virtually no effective computer-based sup-

25

port of an integrative view of patient data [C1O1]. Care providers had to flip among many screens and often among many systems to access data; in some cases, care providers found it easier to manage patient information printed or written on paper.

A reviewer of this report in draft form noted the non-intuitive behavior of most health care IT systems and the training requirements that result from that behavior. Hospitals often require 3- or 4-hour training sessions for physicians before they can get the user names and passwords for access to new clinical systems. Yet much of the computing software that these people use in other settings (e.g., office software) adopts a consistent interface metaphor across applications and adheres to prevailing design/interface norms. As a result, there is much less need for training, and the user manual need only be consulted when special questions arise. In contrast, health care IT lacks these characteristics of conventional software packages—a fact that reflects the failure of these systems to address some basic human interface considerations.

The committee also saw little cognitive support for data interpretation, planning, or collaboration. For example, even in situations where different members of the care team were physically gathered at the entrance to a patient's room and looking at different aspects of a patient's case on their individual computers, collaborative interactions took place via verbal discussion, not directly supported in any way by the computer systems, and the discussions were not captured back into the system or record (i.e., the valuable high-level abstractions and integration were neither supported nor retained for future use).

Instead, committee members repeatedly observed health care IT focused on individual transactions (e.g., medication X is given to the patient at 9:42 p.m., laboratory result Y is returned to the physician, and so on) and virtually no attention being paid to helping the clinician understand how the voluminous data collected could relate to the overall health care status of any individual patient. Care providers spent a great deal of time in electronically documenting what they did for patients [C1O3], but these providers often said that they were entering the information to comply with regulations or to defend against lawsuits, rather than because they expected someone to use it to improve clinical care.

These shortfalls are not necessarily for lack of investment; although health care organizations as a whole spend a relatively smaller percentage of their revenues on IT than do other fields such as banking,[1] one organization—a major integrated health care enterprise with yearly rev-

---

[1]David W. Bates, "The Quality Case for Information Technology in Healthcare," *BMC Medical Informatics and Decision Making* 2:7, 2002, available at http://www.biomedcentral.com/1472-6947/2/7.

enue in the billions—that the committee visited had invested over a half-billion dollars in IT in the past decade. The health care organizations visited demonstrated both deep and sustained organizational and financial commitment to using information technology to improve health care. Yet their health care IT implementation time lines are measured in decades, and it is common to see the implementation of a new generation of health care IT begin while rollout of the prior generation is still underway [C4O16]. Centralization of management and reduction in the number of systems are the predominant method for standardization [C4O15], whereas innovation requires systems that can adapt to local needs [C6O25]. System response times are often slow and long downtimes are common [C4O18].

Consistent with many other reports,[2] the committee recognizes commitment to 21st century use of IT in health care as an essential part of achieving the IOM's vision of 21st century health care. But health care IT is merely a means to the desired end, namely better and/or less expensive health care. The committee believes that clinicians and other providers will, appropriately, be drawn to IT only if, where, and when it can be shown to enable them to do their jobs more effectively. Blanket promotion of IT adoption where benefits are not clear or are oversold will only waste resources and sour clinicians on the true potential of health care IT.

In short, the nation faces a health care IT chasm that is analogous to the quality chasm highlighted by the IOM over the past decade. In the quality domain, various improvement efforts have failed to improve health care outcomes, and have sometimes even done more harm than good.[3] Similarly, based on an examination of the multiple sources of evidence described above and viewing them from the committee's perspective, the committee believes that the nation faces the same risk with health care IT—that current efforts aimed at the nationwide deployment of health care IT will not be sufficient to achieve the vision of 21st century health care, and may even set back the cause if these efforts continue wholly without change from their present course. Success in this regard

---

[2]See, for example, Institute of Medicine, *Crossing the Quality Chasm: A New Health System for the 21st Century*, National Academy Press, Washington, D.C., 2001; President's Information Technology Advisory Committee, *Revolutionizing Health Care Through Information Technology*, National Coordination Office for Networking and Information Technology, Washington, D.C., 2004, available at http://www.nitrd.gov/pitac/reports/20040721_hit_report.pdf; Office of the National Coordinator for Health Information Technology, *The ONC-Coordinated Federal Health Information Technology Strategic Plan: 2008-2012*, U.S. Department of Health and Human Services, Washington, D.C., 2008, available at http://www.hhs.gov/healthit/resources/HITStrategicPlan.pdf.

[3]See, for example, the studies of the Dartmouth Atlas Project at http://www.dartmouthatlas.org/.

Box 3.1 Four Domains of Information Technology in Health Care

Motivated by a presentation from Intermountain Healthcare's Marc Probst, the committee found it useful to categorize health care information technology (IT) into four domains:

- *Automation.* Automation is the use of IT to perform tasks that can be repeated with little modification—examples include bar code medication administration, generation of laboratory results, and issuing invoices for payment.
- *Connectivity.* Connectivity begins with physical infrastructure—ensuring base-level electronic connections between various physical facilities so that data can be transmitted electronically. Examples might include high-speed fiber lines and routing capabilities throughout a physical plant, wide-area networks, and the deployment of wireless infrastructure. Connectivity includes interfaces that map data from one system into another. At the highest level, connectivity involves connecting people to systems and to each other.
- *Decision support.* Decision support (DS) involves the use of IT-based applications to provide information at a high conceptual level to clinicians to facilitate or improve decisions made about care. For example, DS can include simple rule-based alerts such as reminders to physicians about possible drug interactions when medication orders are entered. DS can also involve the presentation of information to care providers in ways that make it easier for them to know how to direct their attention—a "dashboard" indicating patient status across an entire ward or for a physician's 50 sickest patients would be an example of DS for presentation. Finally, DS can also refer to statistical and heuristic decision support reflecting an intelligent synthesis of information about the patient, information from the care setting, and biomedical knowledge—for example, a DS system might recommend a particular antibiotic based on the patient's condition and a database of the recent sensitivity of microorganisms to different antibiotics in their hospital.
- *Data-mining capabilities.* Data-mining capabilities use knowledge discovery techniques to analyze various similar or dissimilar datasets to recognize known or unknown relationships. Data mining converts raw data signals into clinical variables and models to provide a rich source for new approaches to evidence-based medicine and personalized care. Examples range from identification of a marker for breast cancer therapeutic response from microarray data, through mining the text literature for little-known drug-drug interactions, to mining multimedia electronic health records to identify a patient's condition from a text note or a change in heart size from a sequence of images, and extracting ideas or relationships from a recent publication in a leading journal and pushing the information to the physicians who are treating patients who may benefit from those findings. Data mining provides many of the inputs needed for decision support.

will require greater emphasis on the goal of improving health care by providing cognitive support for health care providers and even for patients and family caregivers on the part of computer science and health/biomedical informatics researchers. Vendors, health care organizations, and government, too, will also have to pay greater attention to cognitive support. This point is the central conclusion articulated in this report.

So that the nation can cross the health care IT chasm, the committee advocates re-balancing the portfolio of investments in health care IT; adhering to proven principles for success; and accelerating research in computer science, social sciences, and health/biomedical informatics (and concomitant education about each field for practitioners in the others).

Motivated by a presentation from Intermountain Healthcare's Marc Probst, the committee found it useful to categorize health care IT into four domains: automation, connectivity, decision support, and data-mining capabilities. See Box 3.1.

The majority of today's health care IT is designed to support automation, with some investment in supporting connectivity, and little in support of data mining or decision support. Yet the IOM's vision for 21st century health care expects health care IT that is capable of supporting cognitive activities and a learning health care system. These activities are much more about connectivity, decision support, and data mining than they are about automation. The health care IT investment portfolio must be re-balanced to address this mismatch.

4

Principles for Success

Change in the health care system can take two forms—evolutionary change and radical change. In this context, evolutionary change refers to continuous, iterative improvement of existing processes, sustained over long periods of time, that does not depend strongly on new technological capabilities. The Institute of Medicine (IOM) vision of health care as a "learning system" is one of a system *designed* to benefit from evolutionary change. By contrast, radical change means new ways of looking at health problems and revolutionary new ways of addressing those problems. Radical change often involves a new capability such as the advent of antibiotics in the 1930s and developments in genomics and proteomics today. Some of the automatic data recording, use of novel sensors, data mining, and visualization techniques recommended in this report fit the radical, revolutionary mode of change. Other committee suggestions fit the evolutionary, incremental change mode. Any approach to health care IT should enable and anticipate both types of change since they work together over time.

Abstracting from its site visit observations, the experience of its members, and the extant literature,[1] the committee identified principles to

---

[1] For a sampling of the relevant literature, see M. Leu et al., "Centers Speak Up: The Clinical Context for Health Information Technology in the Ambulatory Care Setting," *Journal of General Internal Medicine: Official Journal of the Society for Research and Education in Primary Care Internal Medicine* 23(4):372-378, April 2008; M.R. Jones, "'Computers Can Land People on Mars, Why Can't They Get Them to Work in a Hospital?': Implementation of an Electronic Patient Record System in a UK Hospital," *Methods of Information in Medicine* 42(4):410-415,

guide successful use of health care IT to support a 21st century vision of health care. In most instances, these principles are not new—but even "old" principles applied properly in a given field or to a given organization can have the impact and significance of new ones. To place emphasis on the importance of each, the text below categorizes these principles into ones related to evolutionary change and those related to revolutionary change.

4.1 EVOLUTIONARY CHANGE

4.1.1 Principle 1: Focus on Improvements in Care—Technology Is Secondary

The most important principle for guiding evolutionary change in health care is to focus efforts on achieving the desired improvements in health care rather than on the adoption of health care IT as a goal in itself.[2] For example, efforts should be structured around clear health care goals (such as those described by the IOM criteria), and with a transparent understanding of the gap between the existing baseline and goal. Only then should there be a focus on process changes needed to close the gap, and an identification of what technology if any is needed to enable the process changes. If early experience shows that the gap is not closing, process and technology can be adapted until the improvement is achieved. In this approach, health care IT is selected and implemented on an as-needed basis to support iterative improvement, instead of being implemented for its own sake at the outset and then potentially becoming a constraint rather than a facilitator of iterative improvement.

2003; J. Øvretveit et al., "Improving Quality Through Effective Implementation of Information Technology in Healthcare," *International Journal for Quality in Health Care: Journal of the International Society for Quality in Health Care* 19(5):259-266, October 2007; Jane Hendy et al., "Challenges to Implementing the National Programme for Information Technology (NPfIT): A Qualitative Study," *British Medical Journal* 331:331-336, August 6, 2005; Heather Heathfield, David Pitty, and Rudolph Hanka, "Evaluating Information Technology in Health Care: Barriers and Challenges," *British Medical Journal* 316:1959-1961, June 27, 1998; C. Sicotte, J.L. Denis, P. Lehoux, and F. Champagne, "The Computer-Based Patient Record Challenges Towards Timeless and Spaceless Medical Practice," *Journal of Medical Systems* 22(4):237-256, August 1998; J.P. Glaser, "Too Far Ahead of the IT Curve?," *Harvard Business Review* 85(7-8):29-33, 190, July-August 2007.

[2]A similar perspective can be found in Carol C. Diamond and Clay Shirky, "Health Information Technology: A Few Years of Magical Thinking?," *Health Affairs* 27(5):383-390, August 19, 2008.

4.1.2 Principle 2: Seek Incremental Gain from Incremental Effort

An important corollary is to engage in a portfolio of activities, starting with ones that require modest investment and are likely to return perhaps modest, but short-term, visible improvements. If programs can be structured so that small investments yield visible success, stakeholders and the relevant decision makers are more likely to be persuaded to continue along such a path. In contrast, programs that require large initial investments of money, effort, and/or time before exhibiting useful results are difficult to sustain and are often politically vulnerable.

4.1.3 Principle 3: Record Available Data So That They Can Be Used for Care, Process Improvement, and Research

Systematic improvement of health care is data-driven. Therefore, health care providers should aggregate as much data as feasible about people, processes, and outcomes from all sources, acknowledging the never-ending challenge of maintaining reasonable degrees of patient confidentiality in such a data collection effort. Of potential relevance are data about people (e.g., their medical condition and health status, their diet and environmental conditions), processes (e.g., actual health care services received, when, and where with detailed process logs), and outcomes (e.g., clinical and functional status at multiple points in time in multiple different conditions). Even if such collected data cannot immediately be regularized to a common semantic standard necessary for full data interoperability, they are still potentially useful for incremental care or process improvement and for research—future needs cannot be fully foreseen, especially in light of anticipated needs for clinical and environmental data to correlate with personalized genomic data. Moreover, systematic advances in process improvement and knowledge may require collection of new data types that cannot be anticipated today, suggesting the need for a collection infrastructure whose scope can be easily expanded. Automatic recording of actions and interactions at the source will facilitate data capture and is needed to avoid increasing the workload of caregivers and ancillary personnel.

4.1.4 Principle 4: Design for Human and Organization Factors

Providers of health care IT can design systems to support people in doing the right thing—by providing incentives for and eliminating barriers to doing those things. Entirely apart from technology, barriers and incentives can be sociological, psychological, emotional, cultural, legal, economic, or organizational. Human-centered design pays attention to all of these factors as they relate to technical function and form. Such work necessarily involves social scientists who understand real human needs and capabilities, why people err, where workload considerations are essential, and how to develop systems that enhance capabilities, that are understandable with minimal training, and that reduce subsidiary task requirements. The use of health care IT designed in the absence of such input may well lead to greater errors, more stress, and lower productivity.[3] In short, success requires not just technology but also—and perhaps more importantly—social and organizational processes to appropriately take advantage of technology.

4.1.5 Principle 5: Support the Cognitive Functions of All Caregivers, Including Health Professionals, Patients, and Their Families

Organizations investing in health care IT can support the cognitive functions of individuals and organizations as they iteratively adapt roles and work processes. Such support includes analysis of data from practice to identify high-priority improvement opportunities among populations or work processes, analysis of applicable evidence, tools such as order sets for linking evidence into workflow, and aggregation of patient data into decision-centric displays. Importantly, cognitive support needs tend to center on high-level decision making (e.g., diagnosis) for populations, patients, or situations, and tend to span granular transactional tasks such as test ordering or prescribing. Cognitive support is not well served by the task-specific automation systems that make up the majority of today's health care IT.

4.2 RADICAL CHANGE

4.2.1 Principle 6: Architect Information and Workflow Systems to Accommodate Disruptive Change

Organizations should architect health care IT for flexibility to support disruptive change rather than to optimize today's ideas about health care. It is axiomatic that health care will change dramatically into the future. New knowledge will become available—e.g., genomic medicine. Population demographics will change—e.g., more people will be elderly, with a correspondingly different emphasis on different kinds of care. Care ven-

---

[3]See, for example, Yong Y. Han et al., "Unexpected Increased Mortality After Implementation of a Commercially Sold Computerized Physician Order Entry System," *Pediatrics* 116(6):1506-1512, December 2005; also, Ross Koppel et al., "Role of Computerized Physician Order Entry Systems in Facilitating Medication Errors," *Journal of the American Medical Association* 293(10):1197-1203, 2005.

ues will change—e.g., more care will be provided at home, and patients will be required to assume greater responsibilities for care (with the assistance of professional care providers). Policy is likely to change—there will be different payment models or reimbursement rates, for example. Thus, any IT-based infrastructure to support today's health care needs must be designed to accommodate changes in roles and process tomorrow—a point suggesting that architectures based on standard interconnection protocols are much easier to change in comparison to monolithic, tightly integrated all-encompassing systems. Otherwise, even deployment of health care IT successful in solving a problem today could stand in the way of solving tomorrow's challenges.

4.2.2 Principle 7: Archive Data for Subsequent Re-interpretation

Vendors of health care IT should provide the capability of recording any data collected in their measured, uninterpreted, original form, archiving them as long as possible to enable subsequent retrospective views and analyses of those data.[4] Advances in biomedical science and practice will change today's interpretation of data. In addition, advances in computer science and related disciplines will lead to new ways to extract meaningful and useful knowledge from existing data stores allowing re-analysis of pre-existing data to reveal medically significant relationships and correlations that are currently unknown. Perhaps most importantly, the committee believes that the availability of large amounts of data is itself a driver for progress likely to inspire medically oriented research in machine learning, display technology, data mining, and so on.

4.2.3 Principle 8: Seek and Develop Technologies That Identify and Eliminate Ineffective Work Processes

Organizations should seek and develop technologies that allow identification and elimination of ineffective work processes and implementation of new approaches to achieving their purpose. Automation of work processes developed in an era when paper was the medium for communicating and archiving is fraught with cost and unintended consequences. For example, some of the work done within the health care system might be accomplished outside health care by providing support for patients

---

[4]See, for example, Werner Ceusters and Barry Smith, "Strategies for Referent Tracking in Electronic Health Records," *Journal of Biomedical Informatics* 39(3):362-378, June 2006. Some of the technology issues involved in archiving are discussed in National Research Council, *Building an Electronic Records Archive at the National Archives and Records Administration: Recommendations for Initial Development*, The National Academies Press, Washington, D.C., 2003.

to better understand their medications and treatment plans. Redesign of work to take advantage of ubiquitous information access and communication may be much more effective than automating existing work processes in an attempt to eliminate errors and effort.

4.2.4 Principle 9: Seek and Develop Technologies That Clarify the Context of Data

Organizations should seek and develop technologies that present new information in the context of other information available about the patient and relevant biomedical knowledge. The combination of new biomedical technologies, together with increased access to data through health care IT, is increasingly overwhelming health professionals' ability to make sense of individual findings. "Alert fatigue" is an example. New approaches are needed to present information in context so that patterns and choices stand out.

5

Research Challenges

There are deep intellectual challenges where the disciplines of computer science and engineering, health/biomedical informatics, related social sciences, information technology (IT), and health care overlap. Indeed, interdisciplinary work will be necessary to go beyond incremental improvement of existing health care IT or the automation of traditional paper-based workflows. Systematic development of the health care IT-related research agenda is beyond the scope of this brief study, but the committee offers a framework for organizing such an agenda.

It is important to distinguish between a solution to a specific problem in the health care domain and the technology-related efforts needed to realize it. The committee conceptualized the necessary technology-related efforts with respect to two separate dimensions. The first lies along an axis describing the extent to which new, generally applicable research is needed. A second lies along an axis describing the extent to which new research specific to health care and biomedicine is needed. Technology-related efforts can thus be separated into four (2 × 2) quadrants, as illustrated in Box 5.1.[1]

From a research management standpoint, such a clustering is helpful for better understanding the parties needed to undertake any given technology-related research effort, the likelihood of its success, the timescale

---

[1]Conceptually, the segmentation of the domain into these four quadrants is quite similar to the division proposed in Donald Stokes, *Pasteur's Quadrant: Basic Science and Technological Innovation*, Brookings Institution Press, Washington, D.C., 1997.

Box 5.1 A Segmentation of Health-Care-Related Technology Efforts

	General applicability	Health care specific
Relatively clear path forward from existing technologies	**Quadrant 1:** General—applied efforts	**Quadrant 2:** Health care—applied efforts
Advanced research needed	**Quadrant 3:** General—advanced efforts	**Quadrant 4:** Health care— advanced efforts

---

needed to achieve success, the appropriate funding mechanisms, and other such parameters. For example, efforts in quadrants 1 and 3 might be pursued by computer science researchers working in loose cooperation with the health and biomedical informatics communities, whereas efforts in quadrants 2 and 4 would require much tighter coordination and cooperation.

These two dimensions emerge from the observation that health care IT draws on classic computer science challenges such as providing high availability with low system management overhead [C4O18], high data integrity, and a very high degree of usability. Such goals are essential foundations of many IT systems but are especially challenging to achieve in the context of health care IT, given the scale and diversity of the health care establishment and, in some cases, the need to support a large, broad user base. In addition, many benefits of systems often accrue only when they are viewed by researchers and caregivers as sufficiently trustworthy to replace older solutions. At the same time, some problems related to health care IT involve solutions that are highly specific to health care (e.g., developing high-quality devices for human-computer interaction [C1O2] that do not inadvertently help to spread infection as care providers move from patient to patient).

As an illustration of how a solution to a major problem in health care might be decomposed into a technology-related research agenda, consider that most clinicians spend a significant amount of time in documenting the care provided to a patient.[2] One challenge for health care IT would be

---

[2]The committee noted this point in its site visits. And the literature has important examples as well. For instance, a survey of more than 2500 clinical oncologists showed that the amount

the creation of a self-documenting environment in which the necessary documentation could be generated with little or no additional effort on the part of the clinicians [C5O19] (see Section 5.2.5). But making progress toward this goal calls for efforts in all four quadrants of the matrix shown in Box 5.1.

The existing technology and general applications of Quadrant 1 provide a clear path for indexing voice recordings. Speech-to-text transcription is a relatively mature technology for vocabularies of modest size as indicated by the variety of commercial software packages available. Speaker identification is routinely performed using voiceprints of the known participants, the patient typically being the remaining unknown speaker during a clinical encounter, and once a voice recording is transcribed to text, indexing within a known domain borders on the trivial. Full-text transcription today has relatively high error rates that make it unreliable as a basis for making clinical decisions, although as the technology further matures, error rates can be expected to drop.[3]

Another general application is information extraction from discourse analysis—a computer listening to a dialog (or examining a transcript) between two people would be able to make inferences about the topics under discussion. Research in this area would build on work in computational linguistics that dates to the 1980s. For deep information extraction (e.g., linking the conversations to key terms in the medical literature), fundamental research in Quadrant 3 is needed (for example) to understand how to relate concepts embedded in the words themselves to the rich store of background knowledge about the world that informs everyday discourse.

As for health-care-specific applications, there is a fairly clear path using existing technology to develop systems that support patient-supplied documentation or documentation provided by the patient's support system (e.g., family), which would increase the continuity and richness of information available for the clinician, as well as being helpful in dealing with expected future burdens on patients to manage their own care outside traditional health care organizations; this research agenda would fit into Quadrant 2. On the other hand, a system to provide a patient or caregivers with interactive explanations of a disease, particularized by the

---

of time they spend filling out paperwork and documenting patient care has increased more than fourfold over the past 25 years. See S. Mayor, "U.S. Cancer Care Is Worse Due to More Paperwork," *British Medical Journal* 322(7296):1201, 2001.

[3]To be sure, claims regarding the impending maturity of speech recognition have been made for a long time, but as with user customization of interfaces (see Footnote 22), speech recognition is another example of an idea that was difficult to implement with the technology of 20 years ago but now is much more feasible with today's technology and just as important today to pursue.

patient's culture, learning style, value system, education, and life experience, remains beyond the current state of today's science and would fit into Quadrant 4.

Other examples of technology-related research efforts in each of the four quadrants are provided below:

- *Quadrant 1* (General—applied efforts). Adaptation of existing IT and process solutions from other domains and industries, e.g., process and data integration technologies, human-computer interaction technologies, ubiquitous networking technologies, security, search, blogging, and social networking.
- *Quadrant 2* (Health care—applied efforts). Identification of the best examples of coupled health care improvement and health care IT that have been successfully deployed or prototyped, followed by wide deployment of those examples. Use of existing data and process standards to obtain low-hanging fruit, e.g., portals, electronic messaging, disease management dashboards, decision support and reminders, process automation, and so on.
- *Quadrant 3* (General—advanced efforts). Invention of new information technologies that are needed in health care, such as ontology management, systems that help to explain why decisions are made, large-scale machine learning, voice technologies, natural language processing, privacy management for access and data mining, and so on.
- *Quadrant 4* (Health care—advanced efforts). Specific advanced work on advanced ontologies and reasoning in the medical domain, modeling of the human body and the virtual patient, interpretation of medical information to different communities, approaches to learning and improving data quality, aggregation of patient health care information into a trustworthy database with explicit representation of uncertainty [C4O17, C5O23]), and so on.

5.1 AN OVERARCHING RESEARCH GRAND CHALLENGE: PATIENT-CENTERED COGNITIVE SUPPORT

Patient-centered cognitive support emerged as an overarching grand research challenge during the committee's discussions. This section discusses how a research agenda might be assembled, together with representative research challenges, to illustrate the magnitude of the opportunity.

Much of health care is transactional—admitting a patient, encountering a patient at the bedside or clinic, ordering a drug, interpreting a report, or handing off a patient. Yet transactions are only the operational expression of an understanding of the patient and a set of goals and plans for that patient. Clinicians have a "virtual patient" in mind—a conceptual model of the patient reflecting their understanding of interacting physiological, psychological, societal, and other dimensions. They use new findings—raw data—to refine their understanding of their virtual patient. Then, based on medical knowledge, medical logic, and mostly heuristic decision making, they formulate a plan, expressed as an order (transaction), to try to change the (real) patient for the better.

Today, clinicians spend a great deal of time and energy searching and sifting through raw data about patients and trying to integrate the data with their general medical knowledge to form relevant mental abstractions and associations relevant to the patient's situation. As reported by Kushniruk, decision making by health care professionals is often complicated by the need to integrate ill-structured, uncertain, and potentially conflicting information from various sources.[4] These various sources include but are not limited to myriad journal articles; memories from personal clinical experience; clinical guidelines; medical records from a host of providers (often working for different health care organizations); informal observations and thoughts from colleagues; and patient commentary and insights. Efforts to sift the data from this collection of sources force clinicians to devote precious cognitive resources to the details of data and make it more likely that they will overlook some important higher-order consideration.

The health care IT systems of today tend not to provide assistance with this sifting task. Rather, they squeeze all cognitive support for the clinician through the lens of health care transactions and the related raw data, without an underlying representation of a conceptual model for the patient showing how data fit together and which data are important or unimportant. There is little or no cognitive support for clinicians to reason about their "virtual patient." So the health care IT systems force clinicians to a transactional view of the raw data. As a result, an understanding of the patient can be lost amidst all the data, all the tests, and all the monitoring equipment.

In the committee's vision of patient-centered cognitive support, the clinician interacts with models and abstractions of the patient that place the raw data into context and synthesize them with medical knowledge in ways that make clinical sense for that patient.[5] Raw data are still avail-

---

[4]A. Kushniruk, "Analysis of Complex Decision-Making Processes in Health Care: Cognitive Approaches to Health Informatics," *Journal of Biomedical Informatics* 34(5):365-376, 2001.
[5]The notion of putting individual medical facts into an appropriate context is not new, having been described in the literature as early as 1969 (Lawrence L. Weed, *Medical Records, Medical Education and Patient Care*, Case Western Reserve University Press, 1969). Nevertheless, IT has progressed a long way since then, providing a more suitable medium in which to implement such a notion.

able, but they are not the direct focus of the clinician. These virtual patient models are the computational counterparts of the clinician's conceptual model of a patient. They depict and simulate the clinician's working theory about interactions going on in the patient and enable patient-specific parameterization and multicomponent alerts. They build on submodels of biological and physiological systems and also exploit epidemiological models that take into account the local prevalence of diseases. The availability of these models would free clinicians from having to scan raw data, and thus they would have a much easier time defining, testing, and exploring their own working theories. What links the raw data to the abstract models might be called medical logic—that is, computer-based tools examine raw data relevant to a specific patient and suggest their clinical implications given the context of the models and abstractions. Computers can then provide decision support—that is, tools that help clinicians decide on a course of action in response to an understanding of the patient's status. At any time, clinicians have the ability to access the raw data as needed if they wish to explore the presented interpretations and abstractions in greater depth.

One possible framework for future health care IT is depicted in Figure 5.1. This framework, which emerged over the course of the committee's discussions and contrasts with the limited focus of today's health care IT, represents an all-encompassing view of components and interactions among components needed to support the Institute of Medicine's vision of 21st century health care.

Future clinician and patient-facing systems would draw on the data, information, and knowledge obtained in both patient care and research to provide decision support sensitive to workflow and human factors. The decision support systems would explicitly incorporate patient utilities, values, and resource constraints such as those mentioned above. They would support holistic plans and would allow users to simulate interventions on the virtual patient before doing them for real. To carry out orders, clinicians would use transactional systems like today's, but built into the decision support system rather than the other way around. In today's systems, decision support is commonly an add-on to systems designed primarily for transaction processing and does not benefit directly from results of data mining. Rather than having data entered by clinicians into computer systems, the content of clinical interactions would be captured in self-documenting environments with little or no additional effort on the part of the clinicians. (That is, an intelligent, sensor-rich environment would monitor clinical interactions and reduce sensor input to notes that document the medically significant content of those interactions.)

In addition to the research challenges related to modeling the virtual patient and biomedical knowledge are the challenges in modeling and

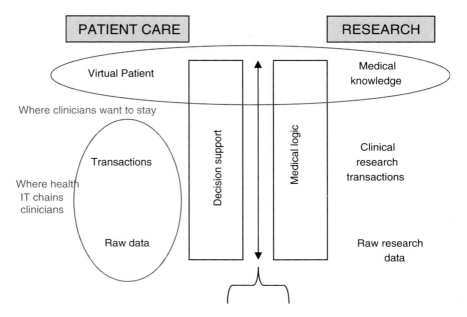

FIGURE 5.1 The virtual patient—a component view of systems-supported, evidence-based practice.

The left side of the figure concerns patient care. Raw data about a patient (the electronic health record) constitute the foundational base. Next come the transactional systems that both produce and use raw data as health care is provided. These two components make up the majority of today's health care IT. Above them, the committee envisions a computational model of the virtual patient.

The right side of the figure represents biomedical science and research and its integral role in health care. Again, raw research data about biological and medical phenomena are at the base. Clinical research transactional systems add to and use raw data during the process of executing or running clinical research protocols. At the top are the models and abstractions that constitute biomedical knowledge. The thread connecting the top three components is what might be called medical logic.

Mapping from medical logic to cognitive decision support is the process of applying general knowledge to a care process and then to a specific patient and his or her medical condition(s). This mapping involves workflow modeling and support, usability, cognitive support, and computer-supported cooperative work and is influenced by many non-medical factors, such as resource constraints (cost-effectiveness analysis, value of information), patient values and preferences, cost, time, and so on.

The virtual patient poses the greatest research challenge but is only one component. Smooth integration with other components is the goal.

supporting multiparty decision making (that is, medical decisions made by family, patient, primary care provider, specialist, payer, and so on). Techniques to interconnect the components are likely to be equally challenging (see, for example, the discussions in Sections 5.2.3 and 5.2.4 on data integration and data management).

Box 5.2 describes some of the technical research challenges for patient-centered cognitive support organized by quadrant.

On the non-technical side, a variety of questions arise as to how the use of clinically oriented systems such as those described above might fit into the actual workflow of a health care organization. How would such support fit into the work patterns of future clinicians? What would the impact be on their work efficiency? How and under what circumstances would clinicians trust the output of these systems? How would responsibility for clinical error be apportioned given the integrative functions of these systems? A failure to answer such questions adequately may well impede clinician acceptance of new approaches, even if the technical challenges can be overcome.

The committee's vision for patient-centered cognitive support is not wholly new. Indeed, development of IT-based tools that examine raw data relevant to a specific patient and suggest their clinical implications was the focus of a great deal of medical expert system work a number

---

Box 5.2 Research Problems Categorized by Quadrant for Patient-Centered Cognitive Support

- *Quadrant 1* (General—applied efforts). Data and process integration technologies, high-quality graphics and sensitive user interface design, coding and application of existing human/health models, application of human language translation technology in some regions
- *Quadrant 2* (Health care—applied efforts). Careful use of existing data standards and models, codification of best practices
- *Quadrant 3* (General—advanced efforts). Reasoning, machine learning, explanation (why the software reaches a particular conclusion), multimodal interfaces (see Section 5.2.5 below); a model of models that would support needed extensibility
- *Quadrant 4* (Health care—advanced efforts). Creation of new advanced models of differential diagnosis; automated machine learning at large-population scale, based on outcomes; a model of models for this domain supporting requisite extensibility

of decades ago.[6] Similarly, biomedical informaticians have worked for decades on the problem of how best to summarize and present data using visual methods, a point of special import in the setting of hospital intensive care units (ICUs), where multiple streams of real-time data can be overwhelming. Much of that research also had to deal with issues of acceptance by ICU clinicians and with trust of the technology.[7] And the importance of connecting biological knowledge to clinical applications has been given new emphasis by a recent focus on translational research by the National Institutes of Health.[8] Nevertheless, the committee believes both that new challenges have indeed emerged and that many "old" problems have proven more difficult to address effectively than was first appreciated. Advances in IT such as the World Wide Web and ubiquitous computing challenge the health care IT community to think differently about how to exploit IT for health care purposes.

A final and significant benefit for the committee's vision of patient-centered cognitive support is that patients themselves should be able to make use of tools designed with such support in mind. That is, entirely apart from being useful for clinicians, tools and technologies for patient-centered cognitive support should also be able to provide value for patients who wish to understand their own medical conditions more completely and thoroughly. Obviously, different interfaces would be required (e.g., interfaces that translate medical jargon into lay language)—but the underlying tools for medical data integration, modeling, and abstraction designed for patient-centered cognitive support are likely to be the same in any system for lay end users (i.e., patients).

---

[6]One of the primary lessons from this work was that although well-designed medical expert systems did have potential to improve clinical diagnoses and recommendations for treatment, many other issues needed to be addressed before they were ready for "prime-time" application. In addition, much of the early work on medical expert systems focused on relatively small problem domains, whereas the overarching medical context for improving health care involves the large problem domain of how all of the patient's data and problems fit together.

[7]See, for example, R.A. Fleming and N.T. Smith, "Density Modulation—A Technique for the Display of Three-Variable Data in Patient Monitoring," *Anesthesiology* 50(6):543-546, June 1979; M.M. Shabot, P.D. Carlton, S. Sadoff, and L. Nolan-Avila, "Graphical Reports and Displays for Complex ICU Data: A New, Flexible and Configurable Method," *Computer Methods and Programs in Biomedicine* 22(1):111-116, March 1986; I.A. Galer and B.L. Yap, "Ergonomics in Intensive Care: Applying Human Factors Data to the Design and Evaluation of Patient Monitoring Systems," *Ergonomics* 23(8):763-779, August 1980; Y. Shahar and C. Cheng, "Intelligent Visualization and Exploration of Time-Oriented Clinical Data," *Topics in Health Information Management* 20(2):15-31, November 1999.

[8]See, for example, Jocelyn Kaiser, "NIH Funds a Dozen 'Homes' for Translational Research," *Science* 314(5797):237, October 13, 2006, available at http://www.sciencemag.org/cgi/content/full/314/5797/237a.

5.2 OTHER REPRESENTATIVE RESEARCH CHALLENGES

In addition to patient-centered cognitive support, there are for the computer science community many other interesting research challenges relevant to health care. Several examples are provided to illustrate this main point, but there are indeed many more that are not covered in this report.

5.2.1 Modeling

One aspect of the "virtual patient" in Section 5.1 involves modeling various subsystems within a real patient (e.g., different organs, digestive system, and so on) to show how they interact.[9] Such models might operate on different or variable timescales—a model focusing on the absorption of nutrients through the digestive system might operate on a timescale of hours, whereas a model focusing on skeletal health, calcium depletion, osteoporosis, or particular bones might operate over years. Similarly, some models might represent molecular interactions, and others might represent particular cells, organs, or organisms.

To first order, the physiological subsystems of all human beings are identical. Thus, a sensible approach to modeling subsystems in a specific patient is to appropriately parameterize a generic model of those subsystems. But finding appropriate parameterizations for any given model and coupling the different models and the data to drive them pose significant intellectual challenges. Some insight into model interoperability can be gained through the use of ad hoc techniques (e.g., XML-based "mash-ups" [Web applications that combine data from multiple sources] used in Web 2.0 applications) or through other existing component frameworks, but the overall problem of model interoperability for health care purposes is vastly more complex than applications that have been tackled before.

Progress is being made in understanding specific metabolic pathways.[10] The effects of a medication, as well as of some other treatments, are candidates for modeling. Such models will still require many of the parameters used to manage and classify the data.[11] Genetic makeup,

---

[9]The notion of a computational virtual human being that would provide a high-fidelity computational model of a human being that would respond realistically to various stimuli is not new. See, for example, "The Virtual Human Project: An Idea Whose Time Has Come?," *Oak Ridge National Laboratory Review* 33(1), 2000.

[10]See, for example, www.HumanCyc.org.

[11]See, for example, PharmGKB, a project to curate information that establishes knowledge about the relationships among drugs, diseases, and genes, including their variations and gene products, available at http://www.pharmgkb.org/.

including the capability to produce pathway-controlling enzymes, is one of the most challenging aspects of making such simulations relevant.

Coupling models will require a computational platform that can support multiple interacting components that can be combined into larger and more complex models. Such a platform must not only support parallel operation of the analytical processes but also allow assembly of hierarchical simulation and information structures, dynamically built, exploited, modified when possible on the basis of individual patient data and statistical aggregates thereof, and abandoned when no longer effective. At the supporting levels, multiple processing alternatives will exist. Specific, detailed simulations will provide the most specific and current results. Cached results can greatly reduce the computational effort for repeated sub-analyses. Where no analytical methods exist, results from biological or clinical trials or clinician assessments can be provided. Search and interpretation can provide yet another set of inputs. Being able to operate with a variety of computational paradigms in one setting can greatly enhance collaboration among communities that have similar objectives but that now ignore each other. Yet another challenge in modeling is building multilevel models that can successfully couple highly detailed physiologic models to the much looser clinical "models" that typically are based more on phenomenological relationships than on true underlying causes.

Finally, keeping records of predictions and actual patient outcomes will allow incremental tuning of the approach. It will take much experience as well as careful approaches to do so in a way that converges on a stable and more optimal outcome. The actual determination of patient treatment will remain in the hands and minds of the clinician. But the feedback that can be provided by bringing data collections, metabolic models, and their processing to an interactive care setting is essential to extract value out of the many technology investments that are in process or being planned.

Box 5.3 describes some of the technical research challenges for modeling organized by quadrant.

5.2.2 Automation

The technical definitions of automation allow for multiple forms, depending on the degree of intelligence and autonomy exhibited. Systems that are completely automatic and that can be trusted to work properly without any need for human oversight or attention have proven to be effective and valuable. Systems that require human oversight or control, which in actuality is almost any complex system, fall under the category

---

**Box 5.3 Research Problems Categorized by
Quadrant for Modeling**

- *Quadrant 1* (General—applied efforts). Development of a framework for easy use of existing, piecemeal models, to gain experience and create a framework for evolutionary advance
- *Quadrant 2* (Health care—applied efforts). Coding and deployment of existing health care models
- *Quadrant 3* (General—advanced efforts). Development of models that self-adapt (or propose self-adaptation) on the basis of changing evidence
- *Quadrant 4* (Health care—advanced efforts). Integration of multiple models, and development of new models

---

of *human-automation interaction* and require considerable care in their design and implementation.[12]

Automatic systems, especially in medicine, do not operate in a vacuum.[13] They are part of a complex network, and the outputs and alarms of automatic systems have to be integrated with other components and often interpreted and, when necessary, overridden by human operators. The intermix of different complex systems plus humans provides widespread opportunity for both good and harm.

Historically, automated systems have often been developed and deployed quite independently of the others with which they must co-exist, leading to confusing and sometimes contradictory signaling, monitoring requirements, and safety concerns. The result is an ever-growing set of alarms (often indistinguishable from one another) and different operating requirements, meaning that new users may not know how to proceed, yet the proliferation of new systems makes it impossible for training to keep apace. The problem of alert fatigue is well known, as evidenced by the

---

[12]For more discussion of this point, see J.D. Lee, "Human Factors and Ergonomics in Automation Design," in G. Salvendy (Ed.), *Handbook of Human Factors and Ergonomics*, 3rd ed., Wiley, New York, pp. 1570-1596, but especially see pp. 1580-1590, 2006; also, T.B. Sheridan and R. Parasuraman, "Human-Automation Interaction," in R.S. Nickerson (Ed.), *Reviews of Human Factors and Ergonomics*, Human Factors and Ergonomics Society, Santa Monica, Calif., 2006.

[13]See, for example, National Research Council, *The Future of Air Traffic Control: Human Operators and Automation*, National Academy Press, Washington, D.C., 1998; National Research Council, *Flight to the Future: Human Factors in Air Traffic Control*, National Academy Press, Washington, D.C., 1997; National Research Council, *The Case for Human Factors in Industry and Government*, National Academy Press, Washington, D.C., 1997.

large number of publications and symposia dedicated to this problem in all industries that are affected: aviation, process control, and medicine.[14]

The worst problem of automatic systems is an issue of trust. If personnel trust them, the trust is often over-generous, so that personnel are apt to believe erroneous indicators and operations for longer than is prudent, or they may neglect attending to and monitoring of the system even though it is not fully reliable. Similarly, a lack of trust may also be inappropriate, leading people to add to their workload to continually check on the operation of a system that is, in fact, quite capable of autonomous operation.

The problems of over- and underautomation have been well documented in other domains and industries, but the committee believes that they have not been appropriately appreciated within the medical community. Much can be gained in an industry by the introduction of more intelligent, more autonomous systems, but the lessons from other disciplines must also be acquired and followed.[15] Automation has been implemented most successfully in aviation and process-control manufacturing. Automation is also used in warehousing and traditional manufacturing, as well as in many modern electronic-commerce back-end systems. Stock trading is another example of an activity in which automation can be used successfully.

All these cases differ from medicine (although prescription filling and checking may come closest to matching order-filling systems), however, and the lessons they provide cannot be carried over directly into medicine. But drawing on such hard-earned experience as a point of departure for medicine makes good sense.

Finally, the introduction of automation is always a systems problem

---

[14]In the medical domain, see, for example, J. Edworthy and E.J. Hellier, "Fewer But Better Auditory Alarms Will Improve Patient Safety," *Quality and Safety in Health Care* 14:212–215, 2005; J. Edworthy and E.J. Hellier, "Alarms and Human Behaviour: Implications for Medical Alarms," *British Journal of Anaesthesia* 97(1):12-17, 2006; A. Otero, P. Felix, F. Palacios, C. Perez-Gandia, and C.O.S. Sorzano, "Intelligent Alarms for Patient Supervision," *Proceedings of the IEEE International Symposium on Intelligent Signal Processing*, WISP 2007, pp. 1-6, 2007.

[15]See, for example, T.B. Sheridan, *Humans and Automation: System Design and Research Issues*, Human Factors and Ergonomics Society, Santa Monica, Calif. (Wiley Series in Systems Engineering and Management), 2002; D.A. Norman, "The 'Problem' of Automation: Inappropriate Feedback and Interaction, Not 'Over-Automation'," in D.E. Broadbent, A. Baddeley, and J.T. Reason (Eds.), *Human Factors in Hazardous Situations*, pp. 585-593, Oxford University Press, Oxford, 1990; C.E. Billings, *Aviation Automation: The Search for a Human-Centered Approach*, Lawrence Erlbaum Associates Publishers, Mahwah, N.J., 1997; D.A. Norman, *The Design of Everyday Things*, Doubleday, New York, 1990; B. Lussier, A. Lampe, R. Chatila, J. Guiochet, F. Ingrand, M.-O. Killijian, and D. Powell, "Fault Tolerance in Autonomous Systems: How and How Much?," in *4th IARP-IEEE/RAS-EURON Joint Workshop on Technical Challenges for Dependable Robots in Human Environments*, Nagoya, Japan, 2005.

**Box 5.4 Research Problems Categorized by
Quadrant for Automation**

- *Quadrant 1* (General—applied efforts). Application of automation systems that exist; more use of business process integration technology as it exists in information technology; application of simple rules that can make a big difference
- *Quadrant 2* (Health care—applied efforts). Codification of low-hanging fruit; use of open-source and other community techniques to pool necessary information to produce better automation rules; application of simple things first, like electronic messaging, automated scheduling of various resources, and so on, and an emphasis on avoiding paralysis by analysis
- *Quadrant 3* (General—advanced efforts). Explanation, self-testing of efficacy, advanced learning, and management of false-negative and false-positive conditions
- *Quadrant 4* (Health care—advanced efforts). Extension of underlying data uses and modeling to improve model precision (e.g., more data feeding into drug interactions systems could be used to reduce false alarms); efforts to ensure that outcomes are known to the system so that it can self-report and learn

---

that intermixes equipment, administrative procedures, and real people. Accordingly, research on automation for medicine will require a multidisciplinary team approach, including technical, medical, and social science expertise. Good design cannot be added on afterward, and intensive cooperative efforts involving people from all disciplines affected by any IT-based system are necessary from the start.

Box 5.4 describes some of the technical research challenges for automation organized by quadrant.

5.2.3 Data Sharing and Collaboration

The data relevant to health care are highly heterogeneous, and the types and quantity of data evolve rapidly. In addition to patient-record information that exists in multiple forms, health care requires data about drugs and diagnoses, including data from signals captured by biomedical devices, voice recordings, and data captured as codes. Data are typically stored in multiple locations on multiple systems. Sometimes such data are stored in structured databases, and in other cases relevant data are found in legacy systems, structured files, and databases and text files behind Web forms. Data are increasingly multimedia and high-dimensional, including voice, imaging, and continuous biomedical signals. Data of various types have different degrees of reliability, ranging from test results (which may be quite conclusive) to patient-provided data (which could contain significant biases). Numerous health care IT challenges require the ability to share and integrate data across multiple systems and seamlessly move data from one system to another.

To exploit highly heterogeneous data effectively, users—such as care-givers, medical researchers, and patients—need the ability to ask queries that span multiple data sources without requiring the data to be stan-dardized or requiring the user to query each single database in isolation. That is, the user wants a single interface through which any query can be posed.

Today, the challenge for data integration, by which is meant systems that enable data owners to share data and collaborate in flexible ways without having to store all the data in a single repository or have them all conform to a common schema, is understood from the systems and logical perspectives. One approach is to aggregate patient health care information into a common data repository [C4O14]. Although aggrega-tion is a basic building block of data integration, aggregating all relevant data into a single repository is likely to be infeasible. As a result of a sig-nificant amount of research, there are commercial systems today that are capable of answering queries that span multiple sources without loading all the data into a single warehouse with a uniform schema. The user of such a system accesses the data through an abstraction called a *mediated schema*, and queries are then reformulated from the mediated schema onto the relevant data sources using a set of *semantic mappings*. These systems perform adequately, and the small additional cost of accessing remote sys-tems at query time is offset by the management benefits of having systems that can share locally owned and maintained components.

The main shortcoming of current data integration systems is that they are too hard to use. Designing a mediated schema and creating the semantic mappings between the sources and the mediated schema entail a significant effort that requires considerable subject-matter expertise. This is especially true when the schema is large, complicated, and likely to be continually evolving, as in the case of health care data. As a consequence, integration projects often fail midway since the costs of this design work are incurred up front before the benefits from that work are obtained.

The above challenge suggests three specific research directions:

- *Data integration systems that are fundamentally easier to use.* The sys-tem should be able to examine the data sources available and suggest to the designers a possible mediated schema and mappings from the data sources to semantically related entries in the mediated schema. The system should point to gaps in the coverage of the data sources so that additional sources can be discovered or enhanced. The system should present to the designer effective visualizations of the data and the schemata to further facilitate the process. Gaps in the system's coverage can be detected by analyzing queries (e.g., frequent queries asking for an attribute of a patient which is not represented in any of the data sources of which the system is aware).

• *Data integration that can proceed incrementally.* It should not be necessary to completely integrate data sources in order to get some benefit from the collection of sources. One approach to reducing the effort required in data integration is what might be called "pay-as-you-go" data integration. A design goal should be the construction of systems that offer access to multiple data sources with little or no human effort, and that improve over time as the users realize where integration is needed most. For example, a system could begin by guessing approximate (and possibly incorrect) semantic mappings; over time, semantic mappings would be improved, thereby enabling more comprehensive answers to queries over the collection of data sources. Some of the specific challenges to obtaining such systems are (1) leveraging user interactions with the system to understand the semantics of the data, (2) developing collaborative techniques for improving the semantic cohesion of a collection of data sources, and (3) maintaining compatibility of incremental integration efforts with previous versions.

• *More flexible architectures for data sharing and integration.* Currently, the common architecture for such systems envisages a single mediated schema and mappings to that schema.[16] While this architecture has the advantage that the data can still remain in the sources and be managed there, the creation of the mediated schema is still a centralized effort. Systems are needed that enable data owners to share data in a more ad hoc fashion and extend the coverage of data sharing as they see fit.[17] Peer-to-peer architectures are needed for sharing data whereby it is easy to (1) discover data sources, (2) join the network of available sources without significant effort, and (3) retain control over the data and its privacy as necessary.[18] In addition, such a system should enable tracking different versions of the data as the data evolve over time, and highlight the changes when appropriate.

If these challenges can be met, it will be much easier to build and deploy data integration systems that require minimal set-up time and pro-

---

[16]See, for example, a common architecture for enterprise information integration products from IBM (http://www-01.ibm.com/software/data/integration/) and BEA (now Oracle) (http://edocs.bea.com/liquiddata/docs81/index.html).

[17]This embodies the philosophy underlying the Semantic Web approach.

[18]See for example, Gio Wiederhold, "Mediators in the Architecture of Future Information Systems," *IEEE Computer* 25(3):38-49, March 1992.

Box 5.5 Research Problems Categorized by Quadrant for Data Sharing and Collaboration

- *Quadrant 1* (General—applied efforts). Application of known data integration technology, ontology management and analysis tools, and state-of-the-art search techniques (including user-machine learning and information retrieval technology to enable systems to self-tune)
- *Quadrant 2* (Health care—applied efforts). Application of existing ontologies and knowledge sources in scalable, efficient systems
- *Quadrant 3* (General—advanced efforts). Development of easier-to-use data integration and ontology management systems, to allow for incremental creation and annotation of semantic information; work toward resolving understanding about how to decide when and where semantics must be added, and when semantics can be induced based on raw information stored and usage models
- *Quadrant 4* (Health care—advanced efforts). Advanced privacy management that supports needs for aggregative, epidemiological research

---

vide valuable services without specifying complete and accurate semantic mappings. For example, certain data regarded as critical might be made interoperable through explicitly designed semantic mappings. But all data might be made available (i.e., visible) subject to control for confidentiality even if no mappings had been created. A care provider needing data for which no mappings were available would have to work harder to query those data, but those data would at least be visible and usable for clinical purposes. If and when a need is recognized for making a particular class of data semantically consistent, mappings could be created—and the system's overall interoperability could be incrementally improved.

Box 5.5 describes some of the technical research challenges for data sharing and collaboration organized by quadrant.

To illustrate the importance of data integration, consider its application to the personal health record. In its ideal future form (not that of today), a personal health record contains an individual's entire medical history, that is, from all interactions with all health care providers (and self-provided care as well) and is under the control of the patient.[19] For information to be easily accessible to the patient, data supplied by different providers—likely each with their own local health care IT systems generating data in idiosyncratic formats and with different meanings—must be integrated in a way that they appear to have common semantics. Data

---

[19]See, for example, Kenneth D. Mandl and Isaac S. Kohane, "Tectonic Shifts in the Health Information Economy," *New England Journal of Medicine* 358(16):1732-1737, April 17, 2008.

protection—a key element of personal health records, in that the patient is empowered to apply fine-grained control of the information contained therein—also requires that patient-specified security and privacy policies act on all data elements referring to the targets of those policies. This requirement presents yet another data integration task.

5.2.4 Data Management at Scale[20]

Presuming the existence of large integrated corpora of data (the focus of Section 5.2.3 on data integration), another major challenge is in managing those data. Some of the important dimensions of medical information management include:

• *Annotation and metadata.* Raw data almost never speak for themselves, and their interpretation inevitably relies on metadata—annotations to the primary data that provide the necessary context. For example, the primary data for the human genome consist of a sequence of some 3 billion nucleotides. Metadata associated with the primary data help scientists to identify significant patterns within those data—a given sequence might be annotated as a gene or a regulatory element. Metadata could also be used to trace the provenance or lineage of data. For example, the value of certain data in an electronic health record could be enhanced if the data included information about the conditions under which certain data were obtained (e.g., physician observations of a patient's description of symptoms might be accompanied by video and audio recordings of the session with the patient). With metadata, a primary problem is the design and development of tools to facilitate machine-readable annotations in large databases.

• *Information extraction from text.* The volume of medically significant information rendered in text form (e.g., physician or nursing notes) is large, and may in various instances be as or more significant than information rendered in different forms (e.g., lab instrument readings). Extracting useful medical information from textual notes is therefore an important problem that calls for computer science expertise in text processing, natural language processing, and statistical text-mining techniques as well as medical expertise to understand the concepts and ideas to which the information refers. New techniques are needed for extracting information such as patient names, doctor names, medicine names, and disease names from textual notes, and for generating automatic linkages between

---

[20]An extended discussion of the data management challenges in biomedical data can be found in National Research Council, *Catalyzing Inquiry at the Interface of Computing and Biology,* The National Academies Press, Washington, D.C., 2005.

different relevant entities. Such extraction would make it possible to piece together a larger picture automatically while pulling information from multiple heterogeneous data and information sources. Extraction of data from tables and figures in reports is another example of a useful information extraction capability.

• *Linkage.* Clinicians often rely on multiple types of data to render a diagnosis—e.g., blood tests and clinical observations and imaging. Relationships between different types of data are best captured in ontologies,[21] which are descriptions of concepts and relationships that exist among the concepts for a particular domain of knowledge. In addition to providing controlled, hierarchically structured vocabularies for medical terminology, they specify object classes, characteristics, and functions in ways that capture important concepts and relationships between those concepts (perhaps in a given area, such as internal medicine or cardiology or oncology). Ontologies containing such information facilitate the representation of working hypotheses and the evidence that supports and refutes them in machine-readable form, and can help clinicians reason their way through complex cases. Ontologies must also be revisable in the light of new research that may discover previously unknown relationships or develop new interpretations of existing concepts. An important research problem is thus the design of appropriate ontologies and automated approaches to populating and updating them through sources such as medical dictionaries, textbooks, and recent articles in the relevant literature, although it is an open question to what extent declarative approaches can capture and exploit all the relevant relationships. Fallback to programmed solutions provides an escape and should be possible to allow putting into practice implementations that can provide feedback and thus enable progress.

• *Privacy.* Epidemiological research and phase IV drug testing (post-approval) both depend on the aggregation of select medical data from large numbers of individual records, even if individual identities need not be associated with these data. The electronic storage of these records facilitates such aggregation, but aggregation on a large scale also has many privacy implications. An important research problem is thus how to mine these data without unduly compromising individual privacy when individuals have not explicitly granted data access permission. Additionally, even outside the world of epidemiological research, the management

---

[21]The term "ontology" is a philosophical term referring to the subject of existence. The computer science community borrowed the term to refer to "specification of a conceptualization" for knowledge sharing in artificial intelligence. (See, for example, T.R. Gruber, "A Translation Approach to Portable Ontology Specification," *Knowledge Acquisition* 5(2):199-220, 1993.)

of data in ways that permit data sharing among those with a need to know, while prohibiting other access, is a significant technical challenge.

• *Scale and other systems issues.* There are many challenges in creating and implementing the protocols and systems that will allow a variety of interlocking systems to provide a robust, high-performance information store that can be reliably and easily accessed by a variety of different classes of users, ranging from the patient and her designees to caregivers. For example, interlocking health care IT systems must enable and preserve the relationships among the different applications and workflows. In addition, the need to store data for a lifetime presents significant technical challenges if only because the storage lifetime could exceed the lifetime of some organizations.

• *User interface.* While technically not data management per se, the data models, data federation technologies, and security and privacy approaches must all support the wide variety of usage that is expected. What an emergency room physician needs is very different from what is required by a physician reviewing the data with an eye toward wellness, a point understood by at least some in the biomedical informatics community since the 1980s.[22] Visualization tools that help users integrate and manage data pulled from multiple sources might also be considered part of a sophisticated user interface, and coupled with analytic techniques may help to solve problems that are not possible to solve using analytic techniques alone.

There are many more dimensions to the problem than those described above, which are intended to be illustrative rather than exhaustive. In addition, Box 5.6 describes some of the technical research challenges for data management at scale organized by quadrant.

In summary, the problems addressed in Section 5.2.3 and in this section are core problems that would lead to the creation of health care records with enormously diverse applications. These applications include providing the information that would, among others things, (1) power the virtual patient described in Section 5.1, (2) provide a strong foundation for epidemiological research, (3) improve communication throughout the caregiver ecosystem, and (4) offer information storage and retrieval that would enable patients and their family and friends to be more involved in their own health care.

---

[22]See, for example, Eric Sherman and Edward Shortliffe, "A User-Adaptable Interface to Predict Users' Needs," pp. 285-315 in M. Schneider-Hufschmidt, T. Kuhme, and U. Mallinowski (Eds.), *Adaptive User Interfaces*, Elsevier, Amsterdam, 1993. User customization of an interface is an example of an idea that was difficult to implement with the technology of 20 years ago but now is much more feasible with today's technology and just as important today to pursue.

Box 5.6 Research Problems Categorized by Quadrant for Data Management at Scale

- *Quadrant 1* (General—applied efforts). Creation of systems that scale, using notions of "cloud" computing, coupled with local information to reduce management complexity
- *Quadrant 2* (Health care—applied efforts). Compression, understanding of what to store and what not to store, prioritization of information; privacy of patient information
- *Quadrant 3* (General—advanced efforts). Techniques for correcting or coding degrees of accuracy and precision in data; techniques for learning about and forming aggregate data sets; automated management techniques for large, highly valuable data sets that are often used across many organizations
- *Quadrant 4* (Health care—advanced efforts). Applications for handling inaccurate data to improve input to health care data models, better coding techniques for information

---

5.2.5 Automated Full Capture of Physician-Patient Interactions

As noted above, care providers spend a great deal of time in documenting their interactions with patients. Automated capture of patient-provider interactions would release such time for more productive uses and help to ensure more complete and more timely patient records.

A comprehensive environment for capturing interactions would necessarily be multimodal, involving ways of capturing and interpreting visual images and conversations. Rather than one general-purpose environment, capture environments would likely be specialized to different settings—such as hospital room (e.g., nurse/patient), emergency room (e.g., ER physician/patient), routine consultation (primary care provider/patient), and specialist consultation (e.g., cardiologist or surgeon and patient).

Some of the important dimensions in this problem domain include:

- *Real-time transcription and interpretation of the dialog between patient and provider.* Individual voices must be identified as being associated with the provider or the patient. The transcript must be parsed unambiguously, irrelevant information identified and ignored, and relevant information interpreted.
- *Summarization of physical interactions between patient and provider based on the interpretation of images recorded by various cameras in the patient care room.* In a hospital room, the system must be able to distinguish

between the administration of an intravenous antibiotic or a tubal feeding. In an examination room, the system must be able to identify parts of the body to which the patient or provider is pointing and correlate such gestures with the dialog. In all settings, cameras should be able to identify documents presented to patients, and to capture written annotations made by patient or provider, subject to appropriate privacy safeguards. The goal would be a system able to produce a useful summary and/or the equivalent of a video transcript that describes what happened.

- *Transcript visibility for patients, and patients' ability to correct and annotate the transcript.*
- *Correlation of the information contained in the audio and visual transcripts.* Use of both types of information should increase the accuracy and utility of the resulting summaries.

Some pieces of this technology exist, but even when they do, integrating them and making the results available smoothly, with little latency, are challenges to today's computer science.

Box 5.7 describes some of the technical research challenges for automated full capture of physician-patient interactions organized by quadrant.

Box 5.7 Research Problems Categorized by Quadrant for Automated Full Capture of Physician-Patient Interactions

- *Quadrant 1* (General—applied efforts). Use of photographic technology, integration of sensor systems (perhaps, from the simple temperature sensor to imaging), use of speech dictation for transcription and/or indexing of audio files, natural language processing on existing textual records
- *Quadrant 2* (Health care—applied efforts). Creation of high-quality workflows, customization of physical devices for the hospital environment (e.g., with due regard for infection control and to minimize physician/patient distance), creation and use of appropriate language models to maximize machine capabilities, workflows to make transcripts available to patients, use of software systems post-visit to provide information
- *Quadrant 3* (General—advanced efforts). Ever-improved speech recognition, multimodal interface development, summarization and extraction of key information, sentiment analysis, automatic privacy management
- *Quadrant 4* (Health care—advanced efforts). Development of new modes of caregiver-patient-computer interaction where the interaction is tri-partite and the computer is not "in the way"; advanced empirical, health care informatics work aimed at understanding how to efficiently acquire and provide information via computer systems

Lastly, a key non-technical issue to be faced by any full-capture system is patient acceptance. In some of today's interactions between clinician and patient, a patient may rely on a clinician's discretion to refrain from entering into the record certain sensitive information related by the patient. In the absence of believable assurances in full-capture clinical interactions that such sensitive information will not be recorded, patients may well be less forthcoming or complete in their accounting of their medical histories and circumstances. Such problems will have to be addressed before any such system will be widely acceptable.

6

Recommendations

Many advances in computer science and engineering in the last 10 to 20 years speak to the problems in health care information technology (IT) observed by the committee. These advances include ontologies, data fusion techniques, large-scale search capabilities, information visualization, and modern computer system architectures to support large-scale distributed systems in a heterogeneous operating environment. But for various reasons, these advances have not often been reflected in generally available clinical information systems.

Organizations face difficult economic decisions regarding whether to emphasize short-term financial gains relative to longer-term advantages wherein cost savings are associated with quality improvement. In addition, the acquisition processes of many health care provider organizations are not often compatible with the development and deployment of future health care IT systems that provide cognitive support and are evolvable into the future. Poorly understood or defined requirements, poor development processes, and failures to adopt iterative or evolutionary approaches or user-centered design are often seen.

In addition, it is fair to say that the integration of health care IT into operational work processes has proven both more essential and more difficult than was first expected, at least in part because many attempts to deploy health care IT have not taken into account the systems engineering issues inherent in viewing health care as a complex, adaptive system. In other words, the research problems have become significantly more demanding when conceptualizing the whole as a set of components working together to provide a working information and knowledge infrastructure for 21st century health care.

Lastly, there are many unsolved problems related to health care IT, including supporting appropriate access while respecting the confidentiality of medical records, managing the cognitive load on care providers that results from the availability of large volumes of information, and managing the information in a medical record over the multidecade lifetime of individuals in the context of rapidly changing scientific and medical knowledge.

Three distinct groups have a meaningful role in addressing these areas. Federal and state government and the health care community must speak to acquisition policy. The health care community must insist that vendors supply health care IT systems that provide meaningful cognitive support. And the research community, including researchers in computer science and health/biomedical informatics, must play a lead intellectual role in advancing the current state of the art in health care IT systems.

6.1 GOVERNMENT

Federal and state governments play important roles as supporters of research, payers for health care, and stimulators for education. The committee believes that government organizations—especially the federal government—should explicitly embrace measurable health care quality improvement as the driving rationale for its health care IT adoption efforts, and should shun programs that focus on promoting the adoption of specific clinical applications. While this principle should not be taken to discourage incentives to invest in infrastructure (networks, workstations, administrative transaction processing systems, platforms for data mining, data repositories, and so on) that provides a foundation on which other specific clinical applications can be built, a top-down focus on specific clinical applications is likely to result in a premature "freezing" of inefficient workflows and processes and to impede iterative change. In focusing on the goal to be achieved, namely better and/or less expensive health care, clinicians and other providers will be eager to use new health care IT-enabled clinical applications if, where, and when such applications can be shown to enable them to do their jobs more effectively.

Health care quality improvement efforts scale from practice groups and individual practitioners to large health care organizations to the health care system as a whole. Traditionally, quality improvement efforts tend to occur at the level of larger practice groups and health care organizations, and are slowed by the requirement to develop consensus among the universe of relevant clinicians. Indeed, these efforts require such volume of collective effort that most organizations cannot sustain more than a few quality improvement initiatives at a time. Given the quality chasm facing many health care organizations, such a slow rate of change is unacceptable.

In contrast, iterative local improvement at the small group or even individual practitioner level has the major advantage of being faster and cheaper to accomplish because of its small scale. This allows for improvement efforts to be conducted in parallel, increasing the chances of finding successful approaches, while unsuccessful approaches can be rapidly and inexpensively discarded. Local successes also tend to build support for additional improvement efforts. Government should promote exploration of methods and models for small-scale improvement efforts as well as efforts to integrate these small-scale improvements on a larger scale. A balance with many small-scale efforts providing the evidence base for a smaller number of large-scale efforts seems appropriate.

IT is a fundamental enabler for both large-scale and small-scale improvement efforts. But for the most part, the health care IT available in today's market is not well suited to support small-scale optimization, which requires applications that are rapidly customizable in the field by end users. Federally inspired or supported initiatives that incentivize health care organizations to undertake iterative small-scale optimization, and subsequent translation of successes to a larger scale, are likely to help stimulate the creation of a new market for these applications—for example, such incentives might take the form of payment premiums for demonstrations of major improvement of a result (process or clinical) for a unit of the organization.

A last point is that work at the health care–IT nexus is interdisciplinary. A lack of familiarity with the domain-specific problems in the health care domain has often impeded the efforts of well-meaning computer scientists. Formal and elegant computer science, as understood by most computer science researchers, is often a poor match with the complex cultural and organizational environment of health care and biomedicine—topics about which a well-trained computer science graduate is generally ignorant. Academic medical centers often fail to take advantage of relevant expertise—especially in health/biomedical informatics—that is available to them. Such organizations are often inclined to turn to internal expertise—the in-house health care IT professionals—rather than to the relevant health/biomedical informatics and computer science faculty on campus. Progress at this nexus will require contributions of health care experts, computer science experts, experts from the health/biomedical informatics community, and health care IT experts working together to understand the problems related to improving health care and how IT might be applied to address those problems.

This analysis leads to six important recommendations for the federal government:

- *Incentivize clinical performance gains rather than acquisition of IT per se.* This is not to say that IT is irrelevant, but the acquisition of health care IT is better guided by what is needed to support improvement efforts.[1] For example, the development and redesign of work processes to provide effective feedback to clinicians logically precede implementation of IT to automate workflow, rather than simply acquiring health care IT first.
- *Encourage initiatives to empower iterative process improvement and small-scale optimization.* Because the market does not today provide the IT required for small-scale optimization (the committee saw no such health care IT in its site visits), these initiatives should also provide support for clinicians to work with computer science and IT experts to design prototype applications to support their improvement efforts. In this short report, the committee did not address the nature or scale of support needed, and believes that this is an issue best addressed in a second phase of this study.
- *Encourage development of standards and measures of health care IT performance related to cognitive support for health professionals and patients,[2] adaptability to support iterative process improvement, and effective use to improve quality.* One lever is to shift the focus of certification efforts from task-specific transactional capabilities to capabilities that provide better cognitive support for health professionals and patients. An example of a standard oriented toward cognitive support would be a requirement to test system effectiveness or human comprehension in the context of the data received by the system or person, perhaps in a simulation environment or in an actual work environment.

---

[1]The federal government has two primary policy levers for promoting an agenda to improve health care quality—public reporting of comparative performance information and pay-for-performance payment policies. Both of these levers depend on the ability to aggregate and analyze data over entire patient episodes, and thus the federal government should require or incentivize submitting the data rather than specifying the particular health care IT to obtain it. Once the data are submitted, their aggregation and analysis can be accomplished through the kinds of health care IT described in Section 5.2.3.

[2]Standards are not a new idea in health care IT—indeed, they are a critical element of "plug-and-play" architectures that enable the infusion of new technologies when they are available (in contrast to monolithic architectures that make it difficult to take advantage of new technologies). However, to the best of the committee's knowledge, standards oriented toward cognitive support essentially do not exist.

- *Encourage interdisciplinary research in three critical areas:*[3] (a) organizational systems-level research into the design of health care systems,
processes, and workflow (i.e., research in systems engineering for a health
care delivery context); (b) computable knowledge structures and models
for medicine needed to make sense of available patient data including
preferences, health behaviors, and so on; and (c) human-computer interaction in a clinical context.

   a. Examples of process and workflow research include languages
   and systems to describe and visualize health care workflows; modeling of health care workflow at scale while enabling explicit step-
   by-step escalation rules; support for distributed, multiplayer decision making among players with sometimes conflicting views of
   what factors are important; rigorous analysis and documentation
   of the workflow demands of routine practice to understand how
   computer technology could be used to facilitate and support the
   workflow of the practitioner; and use of queuing theory to optimize organizational performance.

   b. Examples of research into computable knowledge structures
   and models include computable guidelines and approaches for
   comparing, assessing, updating, and integrating these guidelines
   into a library of guidelines for a given patient; and systems that
   can infer clinical conditions from raw data (e.g., inferring that
   "patient is feeling more pain" from the report of an upward adjust-
   ment in the intravenous drip of a pain management drug). Because
   the clinical interpretation of data depends on the current state of
   knowledge about medicine and about physiology and how people
   respond to treatments and so on, computable structures are important because they connect medical knowledge to patient data in
   machine-readable and machine-executable form. Thus, they can

---

[3]It is beyond the scope of this report to describe in detail the infrastructure needed to
sustain computer science research as it might apply to health care. However, the recommendations from another National Research Council report on research at the interface between
computing and biology are instructive in this regard. That report indicated that

   . . . agencies and foundations should support awards that can be used for retraining purposes;
   balance quality and excellence against openness to new ideas in the review process; encourage
   team formation; provide research opportunities for investigators at the interface who are not
   established enough to obtain funding on the strength of their track record alone; use funding leverage to promote institutional change; use publication venues to promote institutional
   change; support cyberinfrastructure for biological research; recognize quality publicly; recognize
   the costs of providing access to computing and information resources; define specific challenge
   problems that stretch the existing state of the art but are nevertheless amenable to progress in a
   reasonable time frame; work with other agencies; and provide the funding necessary to capital-
   ize on the intellectual potential of 21st century biology. (p. 383)

See Chapter 11, National Research Council, *Catalyzing Inquiry at the Interface of Computing
and Biology,* The National Academies Press, Washington, D.C., 2005.

provide needed abstractions for the health care provider and the clinician to help them understand what is going on with a given patient.

c. Examples of research into clinically oriented human-computer interaction would include the development of systems for maximizing the capture, retrieval, and display of clinically relevant information and handling related uncertainties in ways that minimally distract from attention to the patient and situation yet provide information in a manner that is immediately understandable and interpretable. Such uncertainties include those associated with the information itself and those associated with other matters as well, such as how a patient might respond to treatment or scientific uncertainties about the nature of a disease. Specialized systems would provide different presentations for the different relevant audiences: caregivers, medical staff, insurance companies, patients, and relatives. The research challenge is to be able to extract information relevant to the moment in a way that can readily be assimilated from the tables, graphs, and free-text information about the patient. The collection and recording of information should be incorporated into the normal examination and caregiving actions so that these actions do not disrupt caregiving (as is the case now), yet provide a comprehensive record. Information dashboards would allow a rapid overview of multiple patients, calling attention to cases that require closer examination.

As before, the committee did not address in this short report the nature or scale of support needed and believes that this is an issue best addressed in a second phase of this study.

• *Encourage (or at least do not impede) efforts by health care organizations and communities to aggregate data about health care people, processes, and outcomes from all sources subject to appropriate protection of privacy and confidentiality.* Data aggregation efforts, which should be regarded as infrastructural in nature, will entail some expense, and reimbursement schedules should not discourage such expenses. Recognize that the time for payoff from these systems may be lengthy, while a critical mass of data is being acquired, while data quality is improved, and while systems and processes are developed that can utilize the data. Encourage the decoupling of data from applications (e.g., more reimbursement might be allowed for organizations that have the capability to export data in standard formats that accommodate heterogeneous data types). Where possible, reduce or eliminate organizational and legal barriers to data sharing while taking due note of relevant privacy concerns.

• *Support additional education and training efforts at the intersection of health care, computer science, and health/biomedical informatics*. The purpose of such efforts is to produce more individuals with expertise in both domains—physicians or nurses with undergraduate or graduate degrees in computer science or industrial and systems engineering, computer science researchers knowledgeable about medicine (e.g., with a master's degree in medical innovation) who work on health care problems, and so on. The National Institutes of Health career development programs (often known as the K program) and institutional training programs for medical informatics are models for such support,[4] as are the research training programs in health/biomedical informatics supported by the National Library of Medicine at many educational organizations in the United States.[5]

6.2 THE COMPUTER SCIENCE COMMUNITY

As early as 1992, the computer science community was exhorted to seek intellectual challenges in problem domains of societal significance.[6] Nowhere are such challenges more apparent and important than in health care. Accordingly, the committee believes that the computer science community should:

• *Engage as co-equal intellectual partners and collaborators with health care practitioners and experts in health/biomedical informatics and other relevant disciplines, such as industrial and process engineering and design, in an ongoing relationship to understand and solve problems of importance to health care*. Such engagement will require overcoming important differences of intellectual style that inevitably separate disciplines. For example, there may be intellectual tensions between simplification and abstraction in the service of understanding on the one hand and the capture of details in the service of clinical fidelity on the other—and such tensions will have both positive and negative consequences.
• *Develop institutional mechanisms within academia for rewarding work at the health care/computer science interface*. As argued in other reports,[7] institutional difficulties often arise in academia when interdisciplinary

---

[4]See http://grants.nih.gov/training/careerdevelopmentawards.htm.

[5]See http://www.nlm.nih.gov/ep/GrantTrainInstitute.html.

[6]National Research Council, *Computing the Future*, National Academy Press, Washington, D.C., 1992, available online at http://www.nap.edu/catalog.php?record_id=1982.

[7]See, for example, National Research Council, *Catalyzing Inquiry at the Interface of Computing and Biology*, 2005; or National Research Council, *Fostering Research on the Economic and Social Impacts of Information Technology*, National Academy Press, Washington, D.C., 1998.

work is involved. Collaborators from different disciplines must find and maintain common ground, such as agreeing on goals for a joint project, but must also respect one another's separate priorities, such as having to publish in primary journals, present at particular conferences, or obtain tenure in their respective departments according to departmental criteria. Such cross-pressures and expectations from home departments and disciplinary colleagues remain even if the participants in a collaboration have similar goals for a project. (An example might be the Harvard-MIT program in health sciences and technology.)

• *Support educational and retraining efforts for computer science researchers who want to explore research opportunities in health care.* Such efforts might be offered across a broad front and might span a range in several dimensions, including time and format (e.g., weeks to years; courses, workshops, degree programs, postdoctoral fellowships), content (i.e., different problems within health care), and target audience (i.e., undergraduates to fully tenured faculty).

6.3 HEALTH CARE ORGANIZATIONS

The senior management in health care organizations (including the chief executive officer, chief quality officer, chief medical informatics officer, chief information officer, and chief financial officer) and health care payers have often taken the lead in the deployment of IT for health care and are thus the primary audience to whom the following recommendations are directed.

• *Organize incentives, roles, workflow, processes, and supporting infrastructure to encourage, support, and respond to opportunities for clinical performance gains.* Focus on identifying, prioritizing, and managing changes in process and workflow, and only after doing so support them by technology. Use the context of the organization's quality improvement strategy to guide and correct IT decisions.

• *Balance the institution's IT portfolio among the four domains of automation, connectivity, decision support, and data-mining capabilities.*

• *Develop the necessary data infrastructure for health care improvement by aggregating data regarding people, processes, and outcomes from all sources.*

• *Insist that vendors supply IT that permits the separation of data from applications and facilitates data transfers to and from other non-vendor applications in shareable and generally useful formats.*

• *Seek IT solutions that yield incremental gains from incremental efforts.* Efforts that make progress in many small steps build support and consensus from the grass roots. One example of such an approach might be an institutional commitment to digitize all paper records and make them available electronically in image format to all care providers. Even if capturing paper records in such a form would not make all of their content machine readable, it would go a long way toward eliminating the widely acknowledged problem of record unavailability that plagues a large number of patient-provider visits. And the infrastructure needed for such efforts could be used in the future to support other applications.

7

Concluding Thoughts

The nation has made a commitment to achieve the nationwide use of electronic medical records by 2014. Many meaningful and useful steps can be taken today toward this goal. However, this goal reflects expectations for improvement in the quality and cost-effectiveness of health care that will require more than just wider implementation of today's health care information technology.

At the start of its work, the committee had set out to identify a variety of long-term opportunities for greater involvement of the computer science research community in addressing health care problems. And indeed, the committee did identify a number of such opportunities, which are described above. But it was also struck by the number of other opportunities for meaningful progress that do not depend on research—that is, areas of improvement in which today's information technologies are reasonably adequate for initiating and sustaining meaningful progress and yet are not being fully leveraged for health care. In addition, the committee was surprised to see how little attention had been paid—across the board—to support for the cognitive functions that clinicians use to manage, organize, and coordinate the vast amounts of information needed for effective health care. It is in this domain that the committee believes enormous leaps and bounds are possible, and also where a substantial number of grand research challenges reside.

Appendixes

Appendix A

Committee Members and Staff

COMMITTEE MEMBERS

William W. Stead, *Chair*, is associate vice chancellor for strategy/ transformation and director of the Informatics Center at Vanderbilt University Medical Center. He serves as chief information officer of the Medical Center and chief information architect for the university. The Informatics Center is a unique blend of the units that manage the medical center's information technology infrastructure, the Department of Biomedical Informatics of the School of Medicine (research and education), the Eskind Biomedical Library (knowledge management), and the Center for Better Health (accelerating change). Dr. Stead received his B.A. and M.D. from Duke University, where he also completed specialty and subspecialty training in internal medicine and nephrology. As an undergraduate in the 1960s, he was a member of the team that developed the Cardiology Databank, one of the first clinical epidemiology projects to change practice by linking outcomes to process. As a faculty member in nephrology, he was the physician in the physician-engineer partnership that developed The Medical Record (TMR), one of the first practical electronic medical record systems. He helped Duke build one of the first patient-centered hospital information systems (IBM's PCS/ADS). He led (as principal investigator) two prominent academic health centers, Duke in the 1980s and Vanderbilt in the 1990s, through both planning and implementation phases of large-scale, Integrated Advanced Information Management System (IAIMS) projects. At Vanderbilt, his team has been successful in creating informatics techniques for linking information into clinical workflow, in overcoming the barriers to technology adoption, and in reducing the cost and time required to implement enterprise-wide information technology infrastructure. Dr. Stead is the McKesson Foundation Professor of Biomedical Informatics and a professor of medicine. He is a founding fellow of both the American College of Medical Informatics and the American Institute for Engineering in Biology and Medicine, and an elected member of both the Institute of Medicine of the National Academies and the American Clinical and Climatological Association. He was the founding editor-in-chief of the *Journal of the American Medical Informatics Association,* and he served as president of the American Association for Medical Systems and Informatics and the American College of Medical Informatics. Dr. Stead served as chair of the Board of Regents of the National Library of Medicine, as a presidential appointee to the Commission on Systemic Interoperability, and as a member of the Computer Science and Telecommunications Board of the National Research Council. In addition to his academic and advisory responsibilities, he is a director of HealthStream. Dr. Stead is co-inventor of two patient medical record products—one licensed to McKessonHBOC, Inc., and one licensed to Informatics Corporation of America—from which he receives royalties through Vanderbilt University.

G. Octo Barnett is a professor of medicine at Harvard Medical School and senior research director at the Laboratory of Computer Science (LCS), the clinical and research informatics division of the Department of Medicine at Massachusetts General Hospital (MGH), which provides clinical and research information systems support to the hospital and conducts active research into the application of computer technology in medical record systems, physician workstations, clinical problem solving, expert systems in medical diagnosis, knowledge management, and clinical research. Dr. Barnett's current projects include DXplain®, a decision support system developed at LCS that has the characteristics of both a medical diagnosis aid and a medical reference system; Primary Care Office Insite (PCOI), a focused primary-care-physician-oriented Web site that gathers in a single, easily navigable site a wealth of practical, useful material, including patient care guidelines, therapy information, educational material for patients, and workflow support; and Pulmonary Artery Catheter Waveform Interpretation Tool (PACath), a program that will provide expert knowledge in interpreting and troubleshooting pulmonary artery catheter waveforms. In 1996, Dr. Barnett won the American Medical Informatics Association's Morris F. Collen Award. He is a member of the Institute of Medicine.

Susan B. Davidson joined the University of Pennsylvania in 1982 and is now the Weiss Professor and Chair of Computer and Information Science of the School of Engineering and Applied Science. She is an ACM fellow and a Fulbright scholar, and she recently stepped down as founding co-director of the Penn Center for Bioinformatics (PCBI). Preceding the formation of the PCBI, Dr. Davidson was involved with planning and administering an NSF-funded research training program in computational biology, which has been run at the University of Pennsylvania since 1995. She also helped establish undergraduate degree programs in bioinformatics and computational biology run through the Department of Biology and Department of Computer and Information Science, as well as tracks in this field in the Master's of Biotechnology degree program. Dr. Davidson's research interests include database systems, database modeling, distributed systems, and bioinformatics. Within bioinformatics she is best known for her work in data integration, XML query and update technologies, and more recently provenance in workflow systems. She received the B.A. degree in mathematics from Cornell University in 1978, and the M.A. and Ph.D. degrees in electrical engineering and computer science from Princeton University in 1980 and 1982.

Eric Dishman is the founder, general manager, and global director of Intel Corporation's Health Research & Innovation Group. Trained as a communication scholar and social scientist, Dr. Dishman has used qualitative research methods for more than 13 years to help technology companies understand and invent new market, business, and technology opportunities. He and his team borrow from anthropological and other social scientific methods to interview, observe, and even live with thousands of people around the world at home, work, and play. Dr. Dishman's research has focused primarily on medical anthropology, medical informatics, health care IT technologies, home health care, chronic disease management, telehealth, and aging-in-place technologies, first for Microsoft co-founder Paul Allen, and now for Intel Corporation. As general manager of Intel's Health Research & Innovation Group—part of Intel's newly formed Digital Health Group—Dr. Dishman is responsible for driving global R&D for new health care and wellness-related technologies across the continuum of care from hospital to home. He also directs the Intel Proactive Health Research laboratory focused on home health technologies for seniors and their families who are struggling with cognitive decline, cancer, and cardiovascular disease. Most recently, his group has been conducting pioneering "behavioral biomarker" research by deploying wireless sensor network, digital home, and machine learning technologies into the homes of seniors for unprecedented early detection, differentiation, and personalized treatment of conditions such as Alzheimer's and Parkinson's. Dr. Dishman spends much of his time on the national circuit speaking about and lobbying for new technologies that can help improve health care quality while reducing costs by shifting health care from a reactive, crisis-driven paradigm to a proactive, prevention-driven paradigm. He is a nationally known speaker on the topics of aging and home health care technologies, and he serves as an advisor to numerous companies, universities, and congressional members on assistive technologies, telehealth, and home health care.

Deborah L. Estrin is a professor of computer science with a joint appointment in electrical engineering at UCLA, holds the Jon Postel Chair in Computer Networks, and is founding director of the NSF-funded Center for Embedded Networked Sensing (CENS). She received her Ph.D. (1985) in computer science from the Massachusetts Institute of Technology, her M.S. (1982) from MIT, and her B.S. (1980) from University of California., Berkeley. Before joining UCLA in 2000 she was a professor in the University of Southern California's Computer Science Department. In 1987, Dr. Estrin received the NSF Presidential Young Investigator Award for her research in network interconnection and security. Dr. Estrin has been a co-principal investigator on many NSF- and DARPA-funded projects. She chaired a 1997-1998 ISAT study on sensor networks and the 2001 NRC study on networked embedded computing which produced the report *Embedded, Everywhere*. She chaired the Sensors and Sensor Networks subcommittee of the NEON Network Design Committee. Dr. Estrin is currently a member of the Computer Science and Telecommunications Board and sits on the board of TTI/Vanguard. She is a member of the American Academy of Arts and Sciences and a fellow of the ACM and IEEE, and she received the first ACM Athena Lecturer Award (2006) and the Anita Borg Women of Vision Award (2008).

Alon Halevy is a research scientist at Google, Inc. Before joining Google, Dr. Halevy was a professor of computer science at the University of Washington, Seattle. Prior to joining the University of Washington, Dr. Halevy was a principal member of the technical staff at AT&T Bell Laboratories, and then at AT&T Laboratories. The main goal of his research is to build tools that simplify people's access to data, typically in complex data environments, which he refers to as dataspaces. To support this goal, his areas of research are integrating data from multiple (structured and unstructured) sources, machine-learning approaches to resolving schema heterogeneity, personal information management, management of XML data, and query processing and optimization. He is very interested in the combination of techniques from artificial intelligence and data management. He believes that the data management community should shift its focus away from enterprise computing and consider consumer-facing applications. Dataspace support platforms aim to offer an abstraction at which problems relevant to consumer-facing applications can be addressed. In 1999, Dr. Halevy co-founded Nimble Technology, one of the first companies in the enterprise information integration space. In 2004, Dr. Halevy founded Transformic, Inc., a company that created search engines for the deep Web (i.e., content residing in databases behind Web forms). Dr. Halevy was a Sloan fellow (1999-2000) and received the Presidential Early Career Award for Scientists and Engineers in 2000. He serves on the editorial board of the *Very Large Databases Journal* and on the advisory board of the *Journal of Artificial Intelligence Research*. He served as the program chair for the ACM SIGMOD 2003 Conference and has given several keynote addresses at top conferences. In 2006 Dr. Halevy received the VLDB 10-year Best Paper Award for his work on data integration, and he was elected as a fellow of the Association for Computing Machinery. He received his Ph.D. in computer science from Stanford University in 1993.

Donald A. Norman is the Breed Professor of Design at Northwestern University, where he co-directs MMM, the dual-degree MBA and engineering program offered jointly by Northwestern's schools of management and engineering that focuses on managing products and services from design to execution. He is also co-director of the Segal Design Institute. He is co-founder of the Nielsen Norman Group and has been vice president of Apple Computer and an executive at Hewlett Packard. He serves on many advisory boards, such as the editorial advisory board of Encyclopedia Britannica, and the advisory board for the Department of Industrial Design at the Korea Advanced Institute of Science and Technology (KAIST). He has received honorary degrees from the University of Padova (Italy) and the Technical University of Delft (the Netherlands); the Lifetime Achievement Award from SIGCHI, the professional organization for Computer-Human Interaction; and the Benjamin Franklin Medal in Computer and Cognitive Science from the Franklin Institute (Philadelphia).

Ida Sim is an associate professor of medicine and director, Center for Clinical and Translational Informatics at the University of California, San Francisco. She received her M.D. and her Ph.D. in medical informatics from Stanford University and her primary care internal medicine training from the Massachusetts General Hospital. She is also fellowship-trained in general internal medicine at Stanford University. Dr. Sim's research focus is on knowledge-based technologies for clinical research and evidence-based practice. She received the United States Presidential Early Career Award for Scientists and Engineers in 2000 for her work on the Trial Bank Project, which developed fundamental informatics technologies for a computable knowledge base of randomized trials. She has since led multiple projects related to semantic standards and visualization methods for clinical research, clinical trial reporting bias, new models of scientific e-publication of clinical research, and work on the adoption of electronic health records in primary care practices for quality improvement. In policy work, Dr. Sim was the founding project coordinator of the World Health Organization's International Clinical Trials Registry platform, which sets global standards on clinical trial registration and reporting. Dr. Sim serves on the editorial board of the *Journal of Biomedical Informatics*, is on the advisory board for PLoS One, and is a fellow of the American College of Medical Informatics.

Alfred Z. Spector is vice president of Research and Special Initiatives at Google, Inc. Previously, he was vice president of Strategy and Technology for IBM's Software Group. In other jobs at IBM, Dr. Spector was the vice president of Services and Software Research, the general manager of Marketing and Strategy for IBM's AIM business, responsible for a number of IBM software product families including CICS, WebSphere, and MQSeries, and also the general manager of IBM's Transaction Systems business. Dr. Spector was also founder and CEO of Transarc Corporation, a pioneer in distributed transaction processing and wide-area file systems, and an associate professor of computer science at Carnegie Mellon University. He is an advisor to the Carnegie Mellon School of Computer Science and is a member of the visiting committee of the Harvard School of Engineering and Applied Science. Dr. Spector received his Ph.D. in computer science from Stanford University and his A.B. in applied mathematics from Harvard University. He was the 2001 recipient of the IEEE Computer Society's Tsutomu Kanai Award for major contributions to state-of-the-art distributed computing systems and their applications. He is a fellow of the IEEE and ACM. In 2004, he was elected to the National Academy of Engineering.

Peter Szolovits is a professor of computer science and engineering in the MIT Department of Electrical Engineering and Computer Science (EECS), professor of health sciences and technology in the Harvard/ MIT Division of Health Sciences and Technology (HST), and head of the Clinical Decision-Making Group within the MIT Computer Science and Artificial Intelligence Laboratory (CSAIL). His research centers on the application of AI methods to problems of medical decision making and design of information systems for health care institutions and patients. He has worked on problems of diagnosis, therapy planning, execution, and monitoring for various medical conditions; computational aspects of genetic counseling; controlled sharing of health information; and privacy and confidentiality issues in medical record systems. His interests in AI include knowledge representation, qualitative reasoning, and probabilistic inference. His interests in medical computing include Web-based heterogeneous medical record systems, lifelong personal health information systems, and design of cryptographic schemes for health identifiers. He teaches classes in artificial intelligence, programming languages, medical computing, medical decision making, knowledge-based systems, and probabilistic inference. Professor Szolovits has been on the editorial board of several journals, has served as program chair and on the program committees of national conferences, and has been a founder of and consultant for several companies that apply AI to problems of commercial interest. Professor Szolovits was elected to the Institute of Medicine and is a fellow of the American Association for Artificial Intelligence, the American College of Medical Informatics, and the American Institute for Medical and Biological Engineering.

Andries van Dam has been on the Brown University faculty since 1965 and was one of the Computer Science Department's co-founders and its first chair, from 1979 to 1985. He was a principal investigator in, and director from 1996-1998 of, the NSF Science and Technology Center for Graphics and Visualization, a research consortium including Brown, Caltech, Cornell University, the University of North Carolina (Chapel Hill), and the University of Utah. His research has concerned computer graphics; hypermedia systems; post-WIMP user interfaces, including pen-centric computing, and educational software. He has been working for nearly four decades on systems for creating and reading electronic books with interactive illustrations for use in teaching and research. Professor van Dam received the B.S. degree with honors in engineering sciences from Swarthmore College in 1960 and the M.S. and Ph.D. from the University of Pennsylvania in 1963 and 1966, respectively. He is a member of the National Academy of Engineering.

Gio Wiederhold is a professor emeritus of computer science at Stanford University, with courtesy appointments in medicine and electrical engineering. His recent research includes privacy protection in collaborative settings, large-scale software composition, access to simulations to augment decision-making capabilities for information systems, and developing algebra over ontologies. His current research supports the U.S. Treasury in assessing international intellectual property transfers. Prior to his academic career he spent 16 years in the software industry. His career followed computer technologies, starting with numerical analysis applied to rocket fuel, FORTRAN and PL/1 compilers, real-time data acquisition, and a time-oriented database system for ambulatory care, leading to his eventually becoming a corporate software architect. He has been elected a fellow of the ACMI, the IEEE, and the ACM. He spent 1991-1994 as the program manager for knowledge-based systems at DARPA in Washington, D.C. He has been an editor and editor-in-chief of several

IEEE and ACM publications. Professor Wiederhold served as a contributor and reviewer for several CSTB reports, including *Information Technology Research, Innovation, and E-Government; Youth, Pornography, and the Internet; Technical, Business, and Legal Dimensions of Protecting Children from Pornography on the Internet: Proceedings of a Workshop; Nontechnical Strategies to Reduce Children's Exposure to Inappropriate Material on the Internet: Summary of a Workshop; Review of the FBI's Trilogy Information Technology Modernization Program;* and a letter report to the FBI. Professor Wiederhold received a degree in aeronautical engineering in Holland in 1957 and a Ph.D. in medical information science from the University of California at San Francisco in 1976.

STAFF MEMBERS

Herbert S. Lin is chief scientist at the Computer Science and Telecommunications Board, National Research Council, where he has been the study director of major projects on public policy and information technology. These studies include a 1996 study on national cryptography policy (*Cryptography's Role in Securing the Information Society*), a 1991 study on the future of computer science (*Computing the Future*), a 1999 study of Defense Department systems for command, control, communications, computing, and intelligence (*Realizing the Potential of C4I: Fundamental Challenges*), a 2000 study on workforce issues in high technology (*Building a Workforce for the Information Economy*), a 2002 study on protecting kids from Internet pornography and sexual exploitation (*Youth, Pornography, and the Internet*), a 2004 study on aspects of the FBI's information technology modernization program (*A Review of the FBI's Trilogy IT Modernization Program*), a 2005 study on electronic voting (*Asking the Right Questions About Electronic Voting*), a 2005 study on computational biology (*Catalyzing Inquiry at the Interface of Computing and Biology*), a 2007 study on privacy and information technology (*Engaging Privacy and Information Technology in a Digital Age*), and a 2007 study on cybersecurity research (*Toward a Safer and More Secure Cyberspace*). Prior to his NRC service, he was a professional staff member and staff scientist for the House Armed Services Committee (1986-1990), where his portfolio included defense policy and arms control issues. He received his doctorate in physics from MIT. Avocationally, he is a longtime folk and swing dancer and a poor magician. Apart from his CSTB work, he is published in cognitive science, science education, biophysics, and arms control and defense policy. He also consults on K-12 math and science education.

During this study, **David Padgham** was associate program officer at the Computer Science and Telecommunications Board (CSTB) of the National Research Council. His work comprised a robust mix of writing, research, and project management, and he contributed to the development and publication of numerous CSTB studies. Prior to CSTB, Mr. Padgham was a policy analyst with the Association for Computing Machinery (ACM), working closely with ACM's public policy committee, USACM, to develop and support the organization's policy principles and promote its policy interests. He holds a master's degree in library and information science (2001) from Catholic University of America in Washington, D.C., and a bachelor of arts in English (1996) from Warren Wilson College in Asheville, N.C.

Appendix B

Meeting and Site Visit Agendas and Site Visit Methodology

B.1 MEETING AND SITE VISIT AGENDAS

B.1.1 Meeting 1—April 23, 2007 (Washington, D.C.)

Entirely closed session for NRC housekeeping

B.1.2 Meeting 2—June 13-14, 2007 (Washington, D.C.)

June 13, 2007—Open Session

9:30 a.m.   Welcome
             William W. Stead, Chair
             Jon Eisenberg, CSTB

9:40 a.m.   Charge to the committee
             Donald A.B. Lindberg, Director, National Library of
             Medicine

11:00 a.m.   Panel 1: Health Care IT Industry

             • Industry overview—Greg Walton, Senior VP of HIMSS
               and HIMSS Analytics

- Penetration/adoption gaps, cost, and time to implement—B. Alton Brantley, Consultant
- Untoward consequences—Randy Miller, Vanderbilt University Medical Center

12:30 p.m.   Group discussion and working lunch

1:00 p.m.   Panel 2: Federal Health Care IT Landscape

- Federal landscape—Alicia A. Bradford, Office of the National Coordinator for Health Information Technology
- Commission on Systemic Interoperability recommendations and status—Scott Wallace, National Coalition for Health Care IT
- Standards initiatives—Betsy Humphreys, National Library of Medicine

2:45 p.m.   Panel 3: Visions for Health Care

- Vision for evidence based personalized medicine—IOM EBM Roundtable—Denis Cortese, Mayo Clinic [via videoconference]
- VA's quality transformation: Quality, IT and outcomes— Jon Perlin, HCA
- Vision of a health care system for the 21st century (IOM "Quality Chasm" series, and the challenges in translating visions into practice)—Janet Corrigan, National Quality Forum

June 14, 2007—Entirely closed session for NRC housekeeping

B.1.3 Meeting 3—October 12, 2007 (Washington, D.C.)

11:45 a.m.   Opportunities for improving health care through computer science: Work life of primary care physicians, acute care nurses, and emergency medical technicians
Eric Dishman, Gina Grumke, and Monique Lambert

B.1.4 Meeting 4—January 28-29, 2008 (San Francisco)

Entirely closed session for report development

B.1.5 Online Briefings

November 27, 2007

Peter J. Fabri
Professor of Surgery and Associate Dean, University of
South Florida
Adjunct Professor of Surgery, Northwestern University

November 28, 2007

Peter Neupert,
Corporate Vice President, Health Solutions Group
Microsoft Corporation

December 4, 2007

Kenneth D. Mandl
Assistant Professor of Pediatrics,
Harvard Medical School
Affiliated Faculty, Harvard-MIT Division of Health
Sciences and Technology

B.1.6 Site Visit on September 12-13, 2007
(University of Pittsburgh Medical Center, Pittsburgh)

September 12, 2007

6:20 a.m.   Physician rounds at Children's Hospital of Pittsburgh of
              UPMC
              James Levin

8:00 a.m.   Welcome: UPMC and ISD Overview
              (General information on the number and different types of
              IT systems in use at UPMC, e.g., clinical support systems,
              inventory management, medication management, etc.)
              William Fera
              Sean O'Rourke
              Jody Cervenak
              Ed McCallister

9:15 a.m.   Magee-Womens Hospital of Pittsburgh of UPMC
             overview and demonstration: PPID (Positive Patient
             Identification)
             (Nursing shadowing session)
             Kim Gracey
             Michele Steimer

11:30 a.m.   Children's Hospital of Pittsburgh of UPMC
             overview and demonstration: CPOE (Computerized
             Physician Order Entry)
             (Shadowing session)
             Jacque Dailey
             Steven Docimo
             James Levin
             Jocelyn Benes

2:30 p.m.   Tour of Wiser Institute
             Tom Dongilli

4:00 p.m.   Tour of data center
             Jeff Szymanski

4:30 p.m.   Discussions of UPMC IT systems' technical underpinnings
             Paul Sikora

September 13, 2007

6:30 a.m.   Informal chat session with physicians
             Robert Kormos
             Vivek Reddy

7:30 a.m.   Overview of quality initiatives and Theradoc
             Tami Merryman

9:00 a.m.   eRecord overview
             Daniel Martich

10:00 a.m.   dbMotion and intraoperability
             William Fera
             Sean O'Rourke

12:00 p.m.   Break

2:00 p.m.	UPMC Presbyterian, Physician Rounds Robert Kormos
3:00 p.m.	Adjourn information-gathering portion of meeting

B.1.7 Site Visit on October 10-11, 2007
(Veterans Affairs Medical Center, Washington, D.C.)

October 10, 2007

1:00 p.m.	VistA and patient care services Stanlie Daniels, Deputy Chief Officer, Patient Care Services Mike Mayo-Smith, Chief Consultant, Primary Care
2:30 p.m.	VistA and patient safety Neil Eldridge, Executive Assistant, National Center for Patient Safety
3:30 p.m.	VistA's information technology architecture Joaquin Martinez, Director, Software Engineering and Integration Tracie Loving, Acting Portfolio Management Officer, Management, Enrollment, and Financial Systems
5:00 p.m.	Break and debriefing

October 11, 2007

8:00 a.m.	Chief residents' rounds Medical Service Conference Room
9:00 a.m.	Round with nurse or round with teams Fourth Floor
10:00 a.m.	Greetings and facility overview Fernando O. Rivera, Medical Center Director Director's Conference Room
10:30 a.m.	Electronic health records (EHR), My HealtheVet Ross Fletcher, Chief of Staff Director's Conference Room

12:00 p.m.   Lunch

1:00 p.m.   Surgical admissions nurse
              Admissions Office, First Floor

1:30 p.m.   Emergency room
              Kenneth Steadman

2:00 p.m.   Pharmacy
              Linwood Moore, Assistant Chief

2:30 p.m.   Primary care (Yellow)
              Neil Evans, Co-Chief, Ambulatory Care

3:00 p.m.   Comprehensive nursing and rehabilitation center/
              polytrauma rooms
              Raya Kheirbek, Medical Director

3:45 p.m.   Adjourn information-gathering portion of visit

B.1.8 Site Visit on November 15-16, 2007
(HCA TriStar, Nashville, Tenn.)

November 15, 2007

8:30 a.m.   Welcome and overview of HCA
              Kimberly Lewis, CIO, TriStar Division

9:00 a.m.   HCA information technology systems
              General information on the number and different types of
              IT systems in use (e.g., clinical support systems, inventory
              management, medication management, etc.)
              Annette Matlock, HDIS, Centennial Medical Center
              David Archer, Director, Application Services-Technical
              Darryl Campbell, Director, Application Services-Clinical

10:00 a.m.   Session with content development team
              Melody Rose, Senior Clinical Analyst

11:00 a.m.   Visit medical surgery, ICU
              Kelly Wood, Medical Director
              ICU Nurses

1:00 p.m.   Shadowing session: Doctor(s) on rounds

1:45 p.m.   Shadowing session: Nursing

2:30 p.m.   Observe workflow at a central nursing station

3:30 p.m.   Discussion with chief quality/safety officer
             Ruth Westcott, Vice President of Quality, TriStar Division

4:15 p.m.   Observe workflow at pharmacy/central medication
             management location

5:00 p.m.   Adjourn information-gathering activities for the day

November 16, 2007—Observation Session

8:30 a.m.   Shadowing session: Doctor(s) on morning rounds
             John Wilters, Obstetrics and Gynecology

9:15 a.m.   Shadowing session: Nursing

10:15 a.m.   Observe admissions and/or discharge process (perhaps
             including transition from outpatient to inpatient)

10:45 a.m.   Observe workflow in or take tour of emergency
             department

11:30 a.m.   Informal chat session with a small selection of doctors and
             nurses

1:00 p.m.   Adjourn information-gathering activities for the day

**B.1.9 Site Visit on November 16-17, 2007
(Vanderbilt University, Nashville, Tenn.)**

November 16, 2007

2:00 p.m.   VUMC overview
             William W. Stead, Associate Vice Chancellor for Strategy
             and Transformation

2:30 p.m.   Bed management
             Marsha Kedigh, Manager, VUH Admitting/ED
             Registration

3:15 p.m.   Operating room schedule coordination and technology-
             enabled supervision
             Ken Holroyd, Assistant Vice Chancellor for Research

4:00 p.m.   Pharmacy
             David Gregory, Assistant Director for Education and
             Research, Department of Pharmaceutical Sciences

4:45 p.m.   Demo-process control dashboards and decision support
             Neal Patel, Associate Professor of Pediatrics and
             Anesthesia

5:30 p.m.   Physician work rounds
             Sara Hutchison, Manager, Trauma Unit

6:15 p.m.   Evidence-based content
             Jack Starmer, Assistant Professor of Biomedical Informatics

6:45 p.m.   Nursing shift change
             Sara Hutchison, Manager, Trauma Unit

November 17, 2007

8:30 a.m.   CVICU
             Rashid M. Ahmad, Chief Informatics Officer
             Vanderbilt Heart Institute

9:15 a.m.   Emergency Department
             Corey Slovis, Chair, Emergency Medicine

10:00 a.m.   Architecture
             John Doulis, Assistant Vice Chancellor
             Chief Operations Officer

10:45 a.m.   RHIO
             Mark Frisse, Director, Regional Informatics Program

11:30 a.m.   Biomedical Informatics
              William W. Stead, Associate Vice Chancellor for Strategy
              and Transformation

12:00 p.m.   Adjourn information-gathering portion of visit

B.1.10 Site Visits on December 3, 2007
(Partners, Boston, Mass.)

8:30 a.m.   Brigam and Women's Hospital (BWH)
              John Glaser and David Bates

9:40 a.m.   Overview of BWH inpatient clinical activities: Current and
              future state

10:00 a.m.   General discussion, questions and answers

10:30 a.m.   Tour of the BWH
              Jeff Schnipper and Anuj Dalal
              (Asked to emphasize contact/observation/interaction with
              doctors/nurses)

11:45 a.m.   Tour of central pharmacy and overview of medication
              safety from pharmacist's perspective

1:00 p.m.   Massachusetts General Hospital
              Henry Chueh, Director, Laboratory of Computer Science
              Challenges and opportunities for information
              technology—what has worked at MGH

1:30 p.m.   Ambulatory care practice—Internal Medical Associates
              Blair Fosburgh, Internist, IMA
              What are important issues and opportunities for
              information technology in the practice of medicine?

2:00 p.m.   Carol Mannone, Nurse Leader
              What are important issues and opportunities for
              information technology in nursing ambulatory care?

2:30 p.m.   Virginia Manzella, Administrator, IMA
              What are important issues and opportunities for
              information technology in nursing ambulatory care?

3:30 p.m.   John Goodson, Senior Internist, IMA
               See and discuss the issues and problems of ambulatory
               care practice and the issues and opportunities for
               information technology

4:00 p.m.   Adjourn information-gathering portion of meeting

B.1.11 Site Visit on January 7-8, 2008
(Intermountain Healthcare, Salt Lake City, Utah)

January 7, 2008

8:30 a.m.   Welcome and overview of Intermountain Healthcare, Marc
               Probst, VP and Chief Information Office

9:00 a.m.   Intermountain Healthcare information technology systems
               General information on the number and different types of
               IT systems in use (e.g., clinical support systems, inventory
               management, medication management)
               Stan Huff, Chief Medical Informatics Officer

11:00 a.m.   Introduction to clinical programs at Intermountain
               Healthcare
               Overview of integration of clinical practices with goals,
               direction, and information systems initiatives
               Brent Wallace, Chief Medical Officer

11:45 a.m.   Discussion with chief quality/safety officer
               How are quality, safety, and risk management issues
               addressed at Intermountain? What role does information
               technology play in ensuring quality and safety?
               Lynn Elstein

Observation Session 1   Latter Day Saints Hospital

2:00 p.m.   Latter Day Saints Hospital: Shadowing session: Doctor(s)
               on rounds

2:45 p.m.   Latter Day Saints Hospital: Shadowing session: Nursing

3:30 p.m.   Latter Day Saints Hospital: Observe workflow at a central
               nursing station

4:30 p.m.   Observe workflow in or take tour of ED

January 8, 2008

Observation Session 2—Intermountain Medical Center

8:00 a.m.	Welcome and facility/setting overview
8:30 a.m.	Shadowing session: Doctor(s) on rounds
9:15 a.m.	Shadowing session: Nursing
10:00 a.m.	Observe workflow at pharmacy/drug dispensary/central medication management location
10:45 a.m.	Session with content development team (e.g., order sets)
11:30 a.m.	Informal chat session with a small selection of doctors and nurses Topics include quality, safety, technology, technology implementation, technology's effects on workflow and patient care, and so on
12:30 p.m.	Adjourn information-gathering activities for the day

B.1.12 Site Visit on January 14, 2008 (UCSF, San Francisco)

8:00 a.m.	UCSF, Mount Zion Campus, Women's Health Center Introduction, overview, and quick tour Jon Showstack, Michael Kamerick
8:30 a.m.	Regulatory overhead in clinical research Jon Showstack • Extent and complexity of regulatory overhead of clinical research • Clinical health research considerations (Sharon Friend, Deborah Yano-Fong)
9:30 a.m.	Lack of integration of EMR and clinical research Gail Harden
10:45 a.m.	San Francisco General Hospital Brief introduction and tour of SFGH neurosurgical ICU Geoff Manley

11:00 a.m.   Complexity of data and metadata for querying across heterogeneous databases, especially for translational research
Geoff Manley

B.1.13 Site Visit on January 14, 2008
(PAMF, Palo Alto, California)

12:35 p.m.   Palo Alto Medical Foundation
Welcome and introductions (including working lunch)
Paul Tang

1:00 p.m.   Walk-through of ambulatory care setting
Steve Hansen

1:30 p.m.   Discussion of physician workflow challenges in EHR implementation
Paul Tang, Albert Chan, Charlotte Mitchell

2:30 p.m.   Pitfalls of deriving quality measures from EHRs
Paul Tang, Tomas Moran

3:45 p.m.   Billing and administrative costs from care
Gil Radtke, Neil Knutsen

4:15 p.m.   General discussion

4:45 p.m.   Adjourn information-gathering portion of meeting

B.2 SITE VISIT METHODOLOGY

For each site visit, the committee sought to:

- Observe the best of what the site had been able to achieve.
- Ask about what the site needed but did not have.
- Obtain site input on the gap between needs and the state of the art of the health care information technology industry.
- Identify, clarify, and categorize "pain points" for the site.
- Identify where improvement is possible through application of existing knowledge and where further research is needed.

To preserve face time for interactive questions and answers, each site host was asked to provide as much background as possible as pre-visit reading material. Hosts were requested to limit formal presentations to a

10-minute overview of their key messages, leaving the majority of each time block for interactive exploration. Where possible, hosts arranged for committee visitors to shadow care providers engaged in workday activities (e.g., on rounds, at the central nursing station). Shadowing teams were generally composed of one health care provider and one computer scientist (and one staff person), so that teams could operate in parallel.

Information requested in pre-visit reading material included:

- Organization "facts" (FTEs, admissions, visits, research dollars, and so on)
- Health care organization's organizational chart
- Health care organization's strategic plan
- IT organization chart
- Information management or IT strategic plan
- Information system inventory
- Information technology architecture or standards specifications
- Most recent wired survey responses
- Last joint commission visit report

During each visit, the committee visitors sought to see or to hear about as many of the following facility components as possible:

- Enterprise overview
- IT/systems overview
- Question and answer sessions
  —Chief quality/safety officer
  —Risk management
- Observation points
  —Transition points
    –Bed control, transfer center, life flight
    –Emergency room to inpatient, outpatient to operating room to intensive care unit to intermediate care
    –Medication reconciliation, outpatient to inpatient to outpatient
    –Nursing shift change, house officer signout
- Settings
  —Shadow a nurse during medication administration
  —Shadow a doctor on morning rounds
  —Pharmacy
  —Inventory management
  —Eligibility/billing
- Content management
  —Charge master, reimbursement contracts
  —Formulary, drug-drug interactions
  —Order sets, pathways

Appendix C

Observations, Consequences, and Opportunities: The Site Visits of the Committee

Table C.1, which summarizes the committee's observations from the site visits, is structured as follows.

- **Column 1—Observations (what committee members saw during the site visits).** Under each observation are listed one or more de-identified data points. The high-level observation is the abstraction for those data points. The committee grouped the observations into six categories:

  —Category 1. The medical record itself—the display, the application, the paper; in general, what the user interacts with directly.

  —Category 2. The health care delivery process—the workflow, what happens when, who does it, how decisions are made, how communication occurs.

  —Category 3. Health care professionals—what they are like, how they react to IT, and so on.

  —Category 4. IT infrastructure and management—the underlying computing substrate and how it is managed.

  —Category 5. Data capture and flow—how data are gathered, recorded, and passed among systems, records, and people.

—Category 6. Change in a sociotechnical system—how to create environments that facilitate large-scale change.

- **Column 2—Consequences (why the observations matter).** For each observation, the committee infers one or more consequences. That is, why do we care about the observation in question? How might it affect health care delivery?

- **Column 3—Opportunities for Action (what we can do about the consequences).** Every observation-consequence pair should provide one or more opportunities for action. Solutions known today but not yet implemented are indicated by an "S" (for short-term) in Column 3; challenges for research, where solutions are not known today, are indicated by an "R" (for research) in Column 3.

In Table C.1, the notation $CxOy$ is used. Cx refers to Category x of the committee's observations as grouped in the table (which lists six categories of observations), and Oy refers to a particular observation as numbered in the table (which includes a total of 25 observations).

TABLE C.1 Committee's Observations from Its Site Visits

Observations—What Committee Members Saw	Consequences—Why the Observations Matter	Opportunities for Action—What We Can Do About It[a]
Category 1. The Medical Record Itself		
1 Patient records are fragmented • Computer-based and paper records co-exist • Computer records are divided among task-specific transaction-processing systems • Users have to know where to look • Individual manually annotated work lists are the norm	• Synthesis depends on intra-team conversation • Problem recognition is left to chance • Team members waste time getting information in the form they want to use	• Techniques to synthesize and summarize information about the patient in and across systems with drill-downs for detail (S/R) • Mechanisms to focus on a constellation of related factors (S/R) • Single search box that returns all appropriate information in the appropriate format (R) • Alerts to problems or trends for investigation (S/R) • "Virtual patient" displays leveraging biological and disease models to reduce multiple data inputs to intelligent summaries of key human systems (R)
2 Clinical user interfaces mimic their paper predecessors • The flow sheet is the predominant display construct • No standardization of location of information or use of symbols and color • Font size is challenging	• Important information and trends are easily overlooked • Cognitive burden of absorbing the information detracts from thinking about what the information means	• Design reflecting human and safety factors (S) • Automatic capture and use of context (what, who, when. . .) (S) • Techniques to represent and capture data at multiple levels of abstraction (Care—plan, order, charting; data—raw signal, concept derived from the signal; biology) (S/R)

continued

TABLE C.1 Continued

Observations—What Committee Members Saw	Consequences—Why the Observations Matter	Opportunities for Action—What We Can Do About It[a]
Category 1. The Medical Record Itself (continued)		
3 Systems are used most often to document what has been done, frequently hours after the fact	• Missed opportunity for decision or workflow support • Variable completeness and accuracy • Redundant work	• See Category 5, observation 19 (C5O19)
4 Support for evidence-based medicine and computer-based advice is rare	• Lost opportunity to provide patient-specific decision support	• Peer-to-peer and social networking techniques for development of guidelines and decision support content (S/R) • Mass customization techniques for practice guidelines (modules) (R) • Computable knowledge structures and models (R)
Category 2. The Health Care Delivery Process		
5 High complexity and coordination requirements of care • Within teams • Across teams and services within settings • Across settings	• Reactive care • Handoff errors • Redundant care	• Dynamically computable models to represent plan for care, workflow, escalation, and so on (R)

TABLE C.1 Continued

Observations—What Committee Members Saw	Consequences—Why the Observations Matter	Opportunities for Action—What We Can Do About It[a]
Category 2. The Health Care Delivery Process (continued)		
6 Non-transparent workflow • Clinical roles and responsibilities are not explicit • Scheduling is negotiated and manual • Care processes steps and outcomes are rarely documented in machine-readable manner	• No clear thinking about overall workflows, process design, and efficiency and handoff errors • Unpredictable escalation and response	• Scripting languages for decision and workflow support content (S/R) • Uniform provider ID (S) • Explicit team roles and escalation paths (S/R) • Capabilities for context-aware efficient scheduling (S/R)
7 Work is frequently interrupted with gaps between steps and manual handoffs at seams of the process	• See observations 5 and 6 (C2O5, C2O6)	• See observations 5 and 6 (C2O5, C2O6)
8 Shift of care from inpatient, to outpatient, home, patients, families	• See observations 5 and 6 (C2O5, C2O6)	• See observations 5 and 6 (C2O5, C2O6) • Support for varying cultures and education (R)
9 Errors and near misses are frequent and use of data to identify patterns is rare	• Low voluntary reporting that limits proactive use of near misses for system correction	• Instrumented process to track steps (S/R) • Automated surveillance for potential problems (S/R)
10 Clinical research activities not well integrated into ongoing clinical care	• Difficulty deciding what to charge to whom for research or care • Barriers to subject enrollment • Duplication of research and care processes • Limited learning from routine practice	• Computable models of research plan, workflow, researcher roles, etc. (S/R) • Data exchange between care and research systems (S/R) • De-identification algorithms (S/R)

continued

TABLE C.1 Continued

	Observations—What Committee Members Saw	Consequences—Why the Observations Matter	Opportunities for Action—What We Can Do About It[a]
Category 3. Health Care Professionals			
11	Clinical users choose speed over all else	• Time is money • Each second added to the time to write each prescription in the United States adds 470 physician full-time equivalents	• See Category 5, observation 19 (C5O19)
12	Clinical users do not have a consistent understanding of the purpose of a system or the functionality of the user interface	• Inefficient workflow • Incomplete or inaccurate data entry • Misinterpretation of information • System work-arounds	• Design system modules for use in production (operation) and simulation (training) (S)
13	Health professionals' understanding of how IT might help is limited	• Health professionals do not know what to ask for • Health professionals do not know how to test whether an IT intervention will solve their problem in their setting	• Educate health professionals in systems approaches • Imbed informatics experts in clinical teams (as is done with pharmacists) • Expand informatics training programs

TABLE C.1 Continued

Observations—What Committee Members Saw	Consequences—Why the Observations Matter	Opportunities for Action—What We Can Do About It[a]
Category 4. IT Infrastructure and Management		
14 Legacy systems are predominant • Each is handled as a separate implementation (set-up, profiles, management of decision support content, etc.) • Implementation focuses on the technology, not on enabling process and role changes • Management of change holds all units supported by a system to the implementation rate of the slowest member • Data flow among an organization's systems is very limited	• Rigid workflow in an era of rapid change • Semantic meaning of clinical content is not explicit • Data are not easily shared within or across organizations • Clinical best practice and decision support content are not easily shared	Architectures to permit holistic management of patient information and decision support information across information systems • Decouple infrastructure, transaction processing, data aggregation, and decision/workflow support (S) • Wrap purchased applications as Web services (S) • Leverage ontology and document architectures (S) • Use open-source techniques for infrastructure layer (S) • Develop utility approaches to "operating system on demand" (mass virtualization) (S)
15 Centralization of management and reduction in the number of information systems is the predominant method for standardization	• Does not support a dynamic learning health care system that can adapt to accommodate local needs and capabilities	• See Category 2, observations 5 and 6 (C2O5, C2O6) • See observation 14 (C4O14)

continued

TABLE C.1 Continued

Observations—What Committee Members Saw	Consequences—Why the Observations Matter	Opportunities for Action—What We Can Do About It[a]
Category 4. IT Infrastructure and Management (continued)		
16 Implementation time lines are long and course changes are expensive • Actual implementation time lines for enterprise-wide functionality commonly exceed a decade • New systems are being implemented while the previous generations are still being rolled out	• Requires investment far in advance of benefit • Inconsistent with president's goal for electronic medical records by 2014	• See observation 14 (C4O14)
17 Security and privacy compete with workflow optimization	• Neither is effective	• Techniques to authenticate a patient to his/her record (S/R) • Techniques to loosely couple the individual and his/her identities (S/R) • Architectures that enable confidentiality by limiting access according to need to know while supporting transparency in authorization (S/R)
18 Response times are variable (from subsecond to minutes) and long down-times occur (clinical systems down for >24 hours and equipment down for weeks)	• Work-arounds • Redundant processes • Flying blind	• Approaches that balance local caching of data with timeliness of data (S/R)

TABLE C.1 Continued

Observations—What Committee Members Saw	Consequences—Why the Observations Matter	Opportunities for Action—What We Can Do About It[a]
Category 5. Data Capture and Flow		
19 Data capture/data entry are commonly manual	• More time spent entering data than using data • Variable completeness and accuracy • Loss of opportunity for decision and workflow support	• Redesign roles, process, and technology to capture data at the source as data are created (S/R) • Self-documenting sensor-rich environments (multimedia) (S/R) • See Category 1, observation 2
20 User interfaces do not reflect human factors and safety design • Improperly structured pull-down lists • Inconsistent use of location, symbol, and color	• Systems intended to reduce error create new errors	• Design reflecting human and safety factors (S)
21 Biomedical devices are poorly integrated in every location	• Inefficient charting and intra-team conflict • Inaccurate charting (errors of omission and inappropriate copying) • Unsafe (5 rights errors)	• Mechanism for positively identifying relationship of device to patient and to use (e.g., drip composition) (S) • Handle a physician's drip order (order for substance, titration parameter), the current setting (nurse response to order), and amount actually administered (charting) as three related but separate concepts (S)

continued

TABLE C.1 Continued

Observations—What Committee Members Saw	Consequences—Why the Observations Matter	Opportunities for Action—What We Can Do About It[a]
Category 5. Data Capture and Flow (continued)		
22 Implementation of positive identification technology is problematic • Gaps in the chain of positive identification • Work-arounds are common because of missing or mismatched information • Portable devices are task-specific (different device for lab specimen and medication administration) • Unit doses of medication are not manufactured with computer-readable tags	• Defeats safety objective	• Limit use to subprocesses where the technology is adequate for the workflow (S) • Measure and systematically eliminate work-arounds (S) • Find better technology workflow matches (S/R)
23 Semantic interoperability is almost non-existent	• Lack of interoperability limits data and knowledge reuse	• Interfaces that enable entry of data in flexible ways, but that guide the user into using common fields and terminologies in a non-obtrusive fashion (S/R) • Methods to reconcile multiple references to the same real-world entities (e.g., different ways of referring to penicillin) (S/R) • Mechanisms for mining data to discover emerging patterns in data (S/R)

TABLE C.1 Continued

Observations—What Committee Members Saw	Consequences—Why the Observations Matter	Opportunities for Action—What We Can Do About It[a]

Category 6. Change in a Sociotechnical System

24	Most systems are partially or poorly or incompletely integrated into practice	• Inconsistent use and work-arounds increase error • Benefits are significantly less than anticipated • Reduced investment	• Focus on the desired outcomes instead of the technology (S/R)
25	Innovation requires locally adaptable systems but interoperability and evidence-based medicine require more standardization	• Limited innovation and standardization	• Management that encourages initiation of improvements by health professionals (S) • Technology and processes that allow local innovation and flexibility but foster collaboration and learning at a national scale (R)

[a]R, solutions still to be discovered (research); S, solutions known today but not implemented (short term).